Advance Praise fo
of Santiago Ram

"This is a great addition to the collection of works translated into English of Santiago Ramón y Cajal. The book has two parts. The first deals with several aspects of the scientific career and thoughts of Cajal, in particular regarding his fascination with dreams and hypnosis. The second contains the first English translation of Cajal's dream diary, which provides great insight into how captivated he was by the mental and physiological processes associated with dreams. In 1908 he published an essay about the Theories of Dreaming, in which, he explores the neurobiological interpretation of dreams, reflecting on the question of what the image of the dream is exactly. Thus, the dream diary of Cajal is a theoretical "experimental" approach to his research. In short, this book provides a window through which English readers can enjoy greater access to the intriguing work, and mind, of Cajal."—**Javier DeFelipe, PhD**, Instituto Cajal (CSIC), Universidad Politécnica de Madrid, Madrid, Spain

"Cajal's castigation of Freud's dream theory is as caustic and cogent as his rejection of the reticularist doctrine of a syncytial brain en route to its replacement with his neuron theory. That Cajal kept a dream journal establishes the validity of self-observation for the modern scientific study of the conscious brain-mind." —**J. Allan Hobson, MD**, Professor of Psychiatry, Emeritus, Harvard Medical School, Boston, MA

"Ben Ehrlich delights with a fresh and engaging look at the intricate relationship between two of my scientific heroes. Both were physicians and both tried valiantly to understand the human mind with fundamentally different styles of analysis. It is tempting to conclude that the histologist Cajal—a fervent believer in 'facts'—would have benefitted immensely from a protracted course of Freud's psychoanalysis." —**Larry W. Swanson, PhD**, Appleman Professor of Biological Sciences, Neurology, and Psychology, University of Southern California, Los Angeles, CA

"Santiago Ramón y Cajal, founder of modern neurology and Sigmund Freud, the founder of psychoanalysis who trained as a neurologist, were both captivated by dreams. While Freud made them the road to the unconscious, Cajal, as he dialogued with Freud in a diary of his own dreams, rejected any notion that dreams had meaning. And yet, as Benjamin Ehrlich suggests, so fierce a repression, particularly in the light of images in Cajal's dreams that seem to cry out for a Freudian interpretation, suggests a begrudging acceptance by the neurologist of the very psychological mechanisms whose existence he denied. On another level, reading Cajal's dreams conveys a fascinating and completely novel window into both his biography and the medical culture of Madrid in the early twentieth century."—**Thomas F. Glick, PhD**, Professor Emeritus of History, Boston University, Boston, MA

(continued)

"Anyone who has been inspired by Santiago Ramón y Cajal's scientific brilliance will want to read this sixteen-year record of his dreams, which he transcribed to challenge Freud's theory that dreams are wish-fulfillments. Benjamin Ehrlich's careful translation lets English-speakers explore Ramón y Cajal's dreams, which reveal the vulnerability of one of the world's greatest neuroscientists. In a lucid introduction, Ehrlich lays out the parallels and final divergence of Freud's and Cajal's scientific lives. Do Ramón y Cajal's dreams disprove Freud's dream theory? Readers will have to judge for themselves."—**Laura Otis, PhD**, Emory University, Atlanta, GA

The Dreams of
Santiago Ramón y Cajal

By
Benjamin Ehrlich

Salzburg Global Fellow
Co-Founder, "The Beautiful Brain"
Los Angeles, CA

OXFORD
UNIVERSITY PRESS

OXFORD
UNIVERSITY PRESS

Oxford University Press is a department of the University of Oxford. It furthers the University's objective of excellence in research, scholarship, and education by publishing worldwide. Oxford is a registered trade mark of Oxford University Press in the UK and certain other countries.

Published in the United States of America by Oxford University Press
198 Madison Avenue, New York, NY 10016, United States of America.

Library of Congress Cataloging-in-Publication Data
Names: Ehrlich, Benjamin, 1987– author, translator. | Ramon y Cajal, Santiago, 1852–1934. Suenos. English
Title: The dreams of Santiago Ramon y Cajal / by Benjamin Ehrlich.
Description: New York, NY : Oxford University Press, [2017] | Includes English translation of Los suenos extracted from Los suenos de Santiago Ramon y Cajal / Jose Rallo Romero, Francisco Marti Felipo, and Miguel Angel Jimenez-Arriero. Biblioteca Nueva, 2014. | Includes bibliographical references and index.
Identifiers: LCCN 2016025412 | ISBN 978-0-19-061961-9 (alk. paper)
Subjects: | MESH: Ramon y Cajal, Santiago, 1852–1934. Suenos. | Physicians | Dreams—psychology | Psychoanalytic Theory | Neuroscience
Classification: LCC R690 | NLM WM 460.5.D8 | DDC 610.69/5—dc23
LC record available at https://lccn.loc.gov/2016025412

3 5 7 9 8 6 4
Printed by Sheridan Books, Inc., United States of America

To Marilyn and Alex Ehrlich, with all my love,
and to the legacy of Santiago Ramón y Cajal

CONTENTS

ACKNOWLEDGMENTS

Thank you to Craig Panner for acquiring this book and for your positive feedback throughout the process. It is an honor to publish with Oxford University Press. Thanks also to Emily Samulski for your assistance and to Max Sinsheimer for remembering an old classmate. Thank you very much to Ricardo Martínez Murillo, Fernando de Castro, and Luis Miguel García Segura for generously providing me with the illustrations for this book. I am grateful to the Cajal Institute for preserving and promoting the legacy of Cajal throughout the world. Special thanks to Javier DeFelipe and Juan de Carlos, two of the world's leading experts on Cajal, for encouraging my interest in this material since the beginning and for aiding my project at every turn. Thank you to Miguel Ángel Jiménez Arriero, one of the authors of *Los sueños de Santiago Ramón y Cajal*, for answering my questions about the manuscript, and thank you to J. Allan Hobson for your blessing. Thank you to Thomas Glick, the expert on Freud in Spain, for agreeing to read a draft of my translation and for your ongoing correspondence. Thank you to Elianna Kan for extra translation support and general professional solidarity. I am thankful to Travis Granfar and Bardin Levavy for the patience, generosity, and good humor with which you dispensed your legal counsel.

Thank you to Meehan Crist for acquiring and editing the first excerpts from these dreams for Nautilus and to Michael Segal for publishing my work in your stunning magazine. I am thankful to Susi Seidl-Fox, Salzburg Global Seminar, and all of the fantastic people I met in Austria for that unreal experience. Thanks to S. J. Fowler, Lotje Sodderland, and Thomas Duggan for inviting me over to read and share in London and for facilitating that exciting trip. My deepest gratitude to the Zen Mountain Monastery sangha at the Fire Lotus Temple in New York City for letting me pass through and train in your presence.

My fondest thanks to fellow Cajalians Pablo García López and Virginia García Marín for your kindness and friendship. To Juan Antonio and María Antonia, Ana and Pablo, Tito and Cristina, Angelines and Rafael, Agapito and Marina, Bego, and everyone else: Thank you from the bottom of my heart for the warmth and affection with which you all received me in Madrid. Spending time with your family was among my favorite experiences from my travels. To Marisa: There is no language in which I could adequately express how grateful I am to you. Thank you for taking care of me and for making me feel at home. If not for you, this book would not exist.

I salute and thank all of the terrific minds at NeuWrite in New York City for the distinct privilege of your engagement and critique. My personal thanks to Carl Schoonover, Tim Requarth, Rebecca Brachman, Casey Schwartz, Ferris Jabr, Carl Fisher, and Stuart Firestein for your help throughout the years. Thank you to Carolyn Kuebler, Stephen Donadio, and the estimable *New England Review* for publishing my first translations back in 2012. To Stephen Donadio: I consider myself fortunate that you were and are my teacher. Thank you for your enthusiasm, support, and guidance since the nascent stages of all of this. Thank you to all of my friends in Vermont—more cows than people, more people than I can name. Thanks to Emmanuel "Noah" Hutton, Samuel D. McDougle, and The Beautiful Brain for all your hard work. Thanks to the City and Country School and Word Up Community Bookshop, to my family in Los Angeles and Toronto, and to my encouraging friends everywhere. Thank you to my sister Rachel for letting me play library half the time, and thank you to Jane Parkes for all of your nourishing love and support. Thank you to Mom and Dad for more than I could possibly express in this allotted space, or lifetime.

A NOTE ON THE TRANSLATION

Dreaming in a foreign language is a sign of fluency, but translating dreams from a foreign language can be something of a nightmare.

The act of translation is implicitly fraught with imprecision and compromise, and the dream diary of Santiago Ramón y Cajal presents the translator with a host of limiting challenges. Even if we accept the premise that it is possible to successfully transfer meaning from one language to another, there are still words that defy accurate rendering. For the linguist, these untranslatable words might be appealingly rare and exotic; for the translator, they are nearly impossible to live with or even tame. For example, one of the pet words in this text is *tertulia*, which denotes a distinctly Spanish institution. The term originated in the seventeenth century during the reign of King Philip IV, who was especially fond of the writings of the early Christian polemicist Quintus Septimius Florens Tertullianus, said to be three times the writer that Marcus Tullio Cicero was (thus the epithet Ter for three and tullianus for Tullio).[1] The royal court hosted philosophical discussions in which the ideas of Tertullian were championed; the practice of intellectual debate, which became known as tertulias, spread to the cultural elites. From there, tertulias gravitated to the upper reaches of theaters, where critics would congregate to discuss art and literature in the most comfortable seats in the house. These gatherings then migrated to private residences, until the middle of the nineteenth century, when the tertulia scene became widely popular throughout Spanish cities, staged in cafés and other public sites. By the turn of the twentieth century, tertulias were indispensable to Spanish intellectual life, some eventually evolving into formal academies.

There is no English word that can encapsulate such a storied institution. The closest semantic equivalent for tertulia might be the French word *salon*. However, even if I were translating into French, such a substitution would not suffice because the word salon trails its own historical and cultural associations. Therefore, I have decided to let stand tertulia (as well as *oposiciones*, referring to the inimitable trials in Spanish academia) in the hope that my explanation here provides the necessary context.

In addition to these unique and stubborn creatures is another wild species of words—not untranslatable but multi-translatable—whose ambiguity or vagueness can confuse our comprehension of the text. For example, there are two words in Spanish that mean dream: *sueño* and *ensueño*. Although the two words appear to be almost identical and function in practice as synonyms, their connotations are slightly but significantly divergent. Sueño signifies dream in the narrower sense of mental activity during sleep, whereas ensueño signifies dream in the sense of illusion, vision, or fantasy. Of Cajal's unfinished manuscripts, one was called *Los ensueños* and one *Los sueños*. The distinction between the two words apparently was important enough to Cajal that he petitioned the Academy of Language to distinguish between proper usages. In Cajal's opinion, the ambiguity between these two words made Castilian an inferior language compared to other European tongues. Always the patriot, the language of dreaming was a matter of national pride.

In this dream diary, both Spanish words, sueño and ensueño, appear in the text, most glaringly as headings for different entries. However, there are no two equivalent words in English that are as seemingly impossible to distinguish and yet crucially different in meaning. *Dream* and *hallucination* are not close enough semantically. *Dream* and *daydream* are a perfect match superficially, but technically they are even less compatible because the word daydream limits the experience to the day and daydreams are usually pleasant, whereas ensueños can happen at night and encompass a fuller spectrum of experiences, including nightmares. The word *indream* might be ideal, if such a word existed. In the end, my decision was to render sueño as dream and ensueño as vision, fantasy, or hallucination, even when there seems to be no evidence of Cajal's intention to separate their meanings and when dream for ensueño might work more naturally.

To all native speakers of only English, Spanish is a foreign language, and yet there is another language in this text that is foreign to Spanish and English speakers alike. In theory, cognates should be the simplest words both for the translator to render and for the reader to understand; however, technical vocabulary from highly specialized fields, although shared as a lingua franca among those in the know, is universally inscrutable to everyone else. For example, in the dreams of Santiago Ramón y Cajal, we have the words scaphoid, ganglion, and xylol. In order to know that the scaphoid is a large bone under the thumb, one must be either conversant in anatomy or have had the misfortune to break one's hand; ganglion means a cluster of nerve cells and also serves as a metaphor in Cajal's other writings for primitive organizations of elements of any kind, such as "subordinate ganglionic individualities"; and xylol is a chemical found in certain thinning paints or varnishes but, for histological purposes, serves as a clearing agent to prepare a stained tissue sample for mounting on a slide. These kinds of words can seem at the same time playful and opaque. This text provides some access to the inner voice of a great scientist, which sometimes happens to include snippets of anatomical esoterica. What else might we expect?

Generally speaking, the scientific terminology in Cajal's writing can be vexing, yet there is even more confusion inherent to the medium of this particular work. If dreams are "absurd monsters," then this dream diary is that absurd monster trying to speak. Although there is no standard definition of dreaming, and different fields of study treat the phenomenon fundamentally differently, dream narratives are associated with high degrees of atemporality and bizarreness. The same features, which have thrilled human beings since the beginning of recorded history, make the genre especially confounding to translate. Even when faithful to the dream itself, the dream report will be difficult to comprehend. Dreams are a showcase for the unexpected; the context within which objects appear may be misshapen beyond recognition. For example, the text of one dream entry reads *millones* in one line and *melones* soon thereafter. Although this is likely a typo, it is also not impossible that in a dream about population demographics a melon would suddenly appear.

Necessarily vague and fragmentary, the poetics of dream reporting are usually confounding. However, not many texts are as motley as this; the dreams of Cajal were scribbled on the front and back sides of used sheets of paper and inked in the margins of newspapers and magazines. Given that Cajal's dream report was essentially a collection of notes written by an insomniac, the vagueness becomes opacity and the fragmentation is beyond comprehension. Note writing, a hasty shorthand more permissive of improvisation and abbreviation, is practically its own dialect, showcasing garbled syntax as different from formal writing as night is from day. While Cajal intended to transform this material into a book, the preliminary work was conceived as a private communication, which only he needed to be able to understand; the dreams were not meant to be intelligible to the world. As a direct encounter with unedited thoughts, the experience of reading such a composition is at once psychologically intimate and semantically daunting. We can imagine Cajal, a suffering old man, startling awake or listing in that liminal sea of semiconscious insomnia, perhaps still dazed by a sedative, likely in a great deal of anguish, reaching over to his nightstand to jot down feverishly whatever is in his mind. In such conditions, language tends to degrade, to say the least, and the translator spends most of the time stalled on the lower gear of decoding.

In terms of conventional writing, this text is littered with inconsistencies and errors and pocked with lacunae and omissions. In the ad hoc notation economy, articles are spared, leaving many nouns unspecified. Pronouns are sealed off from antecedents, with multiple claims to possible attachments. Subjects and verbs shun one another in protracted disagreement. This fragmentation, which is inherent to dreams themselves, is exacerbated further by the process of articulation. The material is vulnerable to distortion at every step: During certain phases of sleep, patterns of neuronal activity change and produce signals that are different than those associated with wakefulness. What we experience as dreaming is already an interpretation: The brain somehow translates electrical frequencies into a mental event. The dreamer then records this event, which is another moment of translation. Studies have shown that subjective dream reports are highly variable; for example, according to a 1995 study by John Antrobus, dream reports are twice as bizarre when produced during the late morning than at any other time.[2] The fact is that no one can be relied on to accurately report their dreams, which calls their objectivity into question.

The dream report does not provide direct access to a dream. Its utility as a scientific tool is viewed with skepticism, if it is not dismissed outright. Dream reports seem to fall within the genre of literary translation, with intrinsic patterns of suggestive expression but a highly subjective relationship to the events that they are meant to describe. In the case of Cajal's dreams, the text was further altered through the act of transcription and reproduction, when either Germain or Rallo organized the text in a new form by separating dated dreams from nondated ones and introduced symbols such as [-----], ***, and (?) to indicate Cajal's blank spaces, cross-outs, and illegible words or confusing formulations. It is sometimes difficult to know how certain idiosyncrasies of the text originated. For example, the name of Cajal's friend and colleague appears as Pittaluga in one dream and Pitaluga in another. In fact, Spaniards commonly reduce double consonants that do not exist in their native languages to single. Is this a stylistic choice, an error of transcription, or an original inconsistency? Is it meaningful in the way that Freud suggests in *The Psychopathology of Everyday Life* slips of the tongue or the pen may be? On the whole, the punctuation of the diary can be classified as something between the unorthodox and the negligent. Unfortunately, Cajal's first expressions of his dreams are not available because the original diary no longer exists.

Cajal gave Germain his notes, which Germain typed into a manuscript which he sent, along with the original materials, to Rallo. It is my understanding that Cajal's notes were lost in a flood, but Germain's manuscript survived. In *Los sueños de Santiago Ramón y Cajal*, Rallo describes the physical details of the manuscript, including the yellowed envelope in which it arrived. Rallo had intended to donate Germain's manuscript, which was now the primary source, to the library at the University of

Madrid School of Medicine. However, soon after publishing *Los sueños*, Rallo died, leaving the whereabouts of the text unknown. The sentences are reproduced in *Los sueños* as fragmentary and elliptical, but there is no way of knowing how accurately these editorial choices reflect the original. There is an entry in the diary that reads "(drawing)," and yet there is no drawing to view, nor can we be sure that one ever existed. The greatest challenge in translating the dreams of Cajal is that the text that appears in *Los sueños* has undergone different types of modifications already that have caused an unknowable and irretrievable loss of meaning.

Sigmund Freud considered himself to be a translator; according to Freud, the role of the psychoanalyst was to shepherd preverbal material through symbols past the censor, out from the depths of the unconscious and into the light as meaningful literary narrative. The developmental stages of this text, managed by a psychoanalyst, betrays a classic belief in progression toward understanding. While translating the dreams of Cajal, I found myself gazing in the opposite direction, yearning to regress to the visceral state in which this text was composed. The rawness of the original notes had been neatened by means of mechanical transcription (by Germain) and then reproduced in a more organized form for publication (by Rallo). Every subsequent iteration in this process of refinement destroys the graphological significance of the text, distancing the reader from the emotional and psychological meaning in the act of composition. There would be much to read, if we could see the actual evidence of the way in which Cajal, old, depressed, and gradually enfeebled, moved his pen across the page: the near illegibility of his script, the angling of his lines on the page, the concentration of ink, the dimensions of the blank spaces, the intensity and thoroughness with which he crossed out words, and any accidental markings. Without the preservation and transmission of the text undertaken by Germain and Rallo, the material would have been lost forever. To the extent possible, I have tried to preserve both the semantic integrity of the text and the lack thereof. My sense is that at times the experience of reading dreams of Cajal should reflect their essential incomprehensibility, so as to transmit to the reader the special meaning inherent to the act of composition, now somewhat alienated from the words themselves, yet inescapably suggestive and revealing.

NOTES

1. "Tertulia," Etimología de Chile, www.etimologias.dechile.net/?tertulia.
2. Golos, Lee. "The Stuff of Dreams: A Neurochemical Perspective," Research Gate (2012). http://www.researchgate.net/publication/233969416_The_Stuff_of_Dreams_A_Neurochemical_Perspective.

PART 1

The Founder of Modern Neuroscience

CHAPTER 1

☙

Cajal's Legacy

For all of life is but a dream, and dreams themselves are only dreams.
Pedro Calderón de la Barca, *La vida es sueño*[1]

This book contains the first English translation of the lost dream diary of Santiago Ramón y Cajal (1852–1934), the Nobel Prize-winning "father of modern neuroscience." In the late nineteenth century, while scientific psychologists searched the inner world of human beings for suitable objects of study,[2] Cajal discovered that the nervous system, including the brain, is composed of distinctly independent cells, later termed *neurons*.[3] "The mysterious butterflies of the soul," he romantically called them, "whose beating of wings may one day reveal to us the secrets of the mind."[4] Cajal was a contemporary of Sigmund Freud (1856–1939), whose "secrets of the mind" radically influenced a century of thought. Although the two men never met, their lives and works were intimately related,[5] and each is identified with the foundation of a modern intellectual discipline—neurobiology and psychoanalysis—still in conversation and conflict today.[6] In personal letters, Cajal insulted Freud and dismissed his theories as lies.[7] In order to disprove his rival, Cajal returned to an old research project and started recording his own dreams. For the last five years of his life, he abandoned his own neurobiological research and concentrated on psychological manuscripts, including a new "dream book."[8] Although his intention was to publish, the project was never released. The unfinished work was thought to be lost, until recently, when a Spanish book[9] appeared claiming to feature the dreams of Cajal, along with the untold story of their complex journey into print.

We live in an age of inner space exploration, and the brain is viewed as a final frontier. Since the "The Decade of the Brain"—the 1990s—the promise of "a new era of discovery" in brain research has captivated the public imagination.[10] President Obama recently launched a bipartisan federal initiative to map the human brain, hoping to match the epic success of the Human Genome Project,[11] while the European Union recently granted a billion euros to the The Human Brain Project, the controversial effort to reverse-engineer a functional model of the human brain.[12] Insights into the brain promise to help us treat and cure diseases, design artificial intelligence, and understand the enigma of consciousness. Multiple academic disciplines have attached their names to the end of the prefix "neuro"—for example, neurotheology, neuroeconomics, and neuroliterature ("a division of neurohumanities").[13] Neuroscience is perceived as the new gold standard of intellectual currency. Brain researchers of today have seen their findings inflated, counterfeited, and circulated in self-help books, science-fiction films, web advertisements, and on product labels in every grocery store.[14] That three-pound serving of zombie food turns out to be the most complex object in the known universe. In popular culture terms, the human brain is having a moment.

While this phenomenon might seem like the result of recent trends, the allure of the brain is older than written history. Archaeological evidence suggests that, as early as sixty thousand years ago, European Neanderthals consumed the brain of the deceased during their primordial mourning rituals.[15] Seven thousand years ago, prehistoric humans performed the first neurosurgeries, opening skulls with primitive tools, in an attempt perhaps to revive the dead.[16] The existence of the brain, the meaty pearl of fissured tissue clammed up inside the cranium, has never been in doubt. An organ of the body, as compared with a gene or a particle, the brain is an object of beyond Brobdignagian proportions. The major question in the history of neuroscience has never been whether there *is* a brain but, rather, what the brain does and how. Since Hippocrates declared that the brain is the source of the mind,[17] more than two millennia ago, we have known that what lies between our ears is the essential source material for our entire lived existence. However, despite our timeless obsession with the brain, the general public is not familiar with the visionary man who explored the landscape of our inner world and encountered countless living inhabitants, infinitely small yet largely responsible for our humanity.

Santiago Ramón y Cajal has been called "the father of modern neuroscience."[18] Historians rank him alongside more recognizable names such as Darwin and Pasteur among the greatest biologists of the nineteenth century[19] and Copernicus, Galileo, and Isaac Newton among the greatest scientists of all time.[20] Charles Sherrington, another pioneer of modern neuroscience, called Cajal the greatest anatomist of the nervous system ever known,[21] in full knowledge of the fact that there have been anatomists investigating the nervous system since ancient times. Cajal's groundbreaking work on the structure of the nervous system earned him every conceivable prestigious award, including the 1906 Nobel Prize in Physiology or Medicine. His magnum opus, *The Texture of the Nervous System of Man and Vertebrates*, "one of the masterpieces of the history of science,"[22] is a foundational text for neuroscience comparable to *On the Origin of Species* for evolutionary biology.[23] More than a century later, Cajal's works are cited hundreds of times each year in the scientific literature.[24] The oldest neuroscience society in North America is called the Cajal Club, with more than five hundred members who share a secret handshake.[25] There is more than one neuroscientist in the world right now with an image of one of Cajal's scientific drawings tattooed on her or his body.[26] How many scientists can boast of such a citation? Even those critics who decry Cajal's cult-like following cannot deny his lasting influence.[27]

In his native Spain, Cajal was a national hero. There is a street named after him in virtually every Spanish city.[28] When he died, thousands of people from different social classes mourned him in the royal capital of Madrid. In the midst of a potential revolution, as a union of coal miners continued its premonitory armed resistance against the national military,[29] both the liberal republican and the conservative monarchist newspapers conceded valuable space above the fold to glorify Cajal. His stern, white-bearded, bespectacled face was printed on the fifty-peseta note the year after his death. In the leafy haven of Retiro Park, the Central Park of Madrid, there is a statue of him resting between the symbolic fountains of life and death, draped by a toga, watched over by Minerva, the Goddess of Wisdom. The King of Spain, Alfonso XIII, built the first national biological research facility to support his work. Still renowned to this day, the Cajal Institute participates in a collective Spanish effort on behalf of the Human Brain Project, "Cajal Blue Brain," named for the founder of their proud national tradition.

Historically known for its artists, writers, and conquistadors, Spain became home to an unlikely scientific legend who nonetheless identified with each of those classical archetypes. Cajal was a microscopic anatomist who cast himself as a grand explorer. "The brain is a world," he once said, "consisting of a number of unexplored continents and great stretches of unknown territory."[30] He spent forty years—for an average of fifteen hours every day, in his prime[31]—dissecting organic tissue, staining the samples with chemicals, and staring through the microscope to discern their subtle traceries. This method, known as *histology*, allowed investigators to visualize the finest structures hidden within life on earth. By the middle of the century, biologists had established distinctly individual units—termed *cells* for their resemblance to the living quarters of monks—as the basic units of composition in every organism. The brain, especially difficult to visualize because of its dense concentration of fibers, remained the final exception and a matter of considerable vagueness and confusion.

In Cajal's day, the prevailing scientific theory held that the brain was composed of a reticulum, a continuous tangle of rigid fibers, unnavigable as a labyrinth. There were a few anatomists at the time who challenged this structure. In order to shift the paradigm, however, someone needed to produce convincing evidence of independent cells in the brain, whose fibers were definitively not connected. Working alone, in his makeshift home laboratory, Cajal, a university professor of anatomy, harnessed a powerful and erratic technique that revealed a select number of nerves in their entirety, unusued for over a decade. Guiding himself by their faint, black fibers, he turned the slide and adjusted his focus until reaching the free end of a string. Cajal declared the complete autonomy of the nerve cell in 1888,[32] in the style of a revolutionary. After convincing his peers of these radical findings, the "new truth" started to spread. A few years later, German anatomist Wilhelm Waldeyer, summarizing Cajal's work and the work of his fellow anatomists, named the brain cells *neurons*, from the epic Greek word meaning *tendon*.[33] The neuron theory developed into the final extension of cell theory and remains the foundation of neuroscience to this day. If all Russian literature comes from Gogol's "Overcoat," and all modern American literature comes from a book by Mark Twain called *Huckleberry Finn*, then the tradition of modern brain research comes from the work of Santiago Ramón y Cajal.

One of the keys to Cajal's scientific vision was his special attachment to neurons and cells in general. In his autobiography, *Recollections of My Life*, he describes his first microscopic views of human anatomy as "scenes from life of the infinitely small,"[34] like characters in a miniscule drama. For Cajal, the movement of red and white blood cells was a saga that could grip his attention for twenty straight hours.[35] In his more philosophical early essays promoting cell theory, he pointed out that he, as the observer, was made of the same material as his subject, the single-cell microorganism.[36] Cajal wrote science fiction stories about a human being that shrinks to a microscopic size. Paraphrasing the famous cell theorist Rudolf Virchow, Cajal called the cell "an autonomous living being that is the exclusive protagonist of pathological episodes."[37] The descriptive language that he employs in his investigations of the brain implies a certain spirited agency: The probing ends of growing fibers are *battering rams*, and the fateful meeting between two communicating neurons, later termed the *synapse*, he likened to a *protoplasmic kiss*, "the final ecstasy of an epic love story."[38] Cajal's way of seeing the brain was, thus, intensely anthropomorphic. According to Sherrington, "He treated the microscopic scene as though it were alive and were inhabited by beings which felt and did and hoped and tried even as we do."[39] "If we would enter adequately into Cajal's thought in this field," Sherrington said, "we must suppose his entrance, through the microscope, into a world populated by tiny beings actuated by motives and striving and satisfactions not very remotely different from our own."[40] When Cajal looked into the brain, he imagined neurons as miniature versions of himself.

Cajal studied neurons throughout their life cycles, and his research interests reflect the preoccupations of his own life. His obsession with their youthful independence reflected his own struggles to separate from his family and stand on his own; later, his insistence on their irreversible degeneration mirrored his fears about his own decline. Cajal's particular psychology, the way he projected his own beliefs onto his slides, allowed him to interpret subtle and significant anatomical structures, such as *growth cones* and *dendritic spines*, that his scientific peers often overlooked or dismissed. In *The Texture of the Nervous System*, he travels the nervous system, like the hero from his youthful fictions, classifying and describing the different types of neurons as though they were foreign peoples toward whom he felt a deep affinity. He studied their *morphology* in order to trace their patterns of development, from birth to death. His later work, *Regeneration and Degeneration of the Nervous System*,[41] another classic, considered their responses to trauma and injury. Cajal saw humanity inside the brain, and this was the key to his profound scientific understanding.

In his final testament to the neuron theory, translated as *Neuron Theory or Reticular Theory?*[42] Cajal reported to have seen more than a million neurons. Cajal's drawings of these neurons are much like portraits. After multiple observations of different cells, Cajal would generalize their features into synthesized compositions. At times, he would look through the microscope with one eye, with the other trained on his sketching hand. Depending on the staining method, Cajal used pencil and Chinese ink, adding graphite for relief effects, and watercolors or aquarelles when necessary.[43] According to his own estimate, he produced twelve thousand drawings of the nervous system, or an average of two per day, mostly on the backs of papers or in the margins of letters, notated with instructions for future publication. Even with the invention of microphotography, Cajal preferred drawing his images by hand.

Although some colleagues criticized his methods as overly interpretive, Cajal argued that due to uniqueness of detail in each individual cell, the selection, combination, and even alteration of certain features was necessary to form a coherent and representative image. Despite the subsequent advances in technology and their unimaginable capacities for heightened visualization, these original illustrations regularly appear in textbooks and still are considered to be faithful and accurate, more than a century later. These same illustrations now are starting to receive the attention that they deserve, in books and on museum walls, as works of art.[44] "Only true artists are attracted to science," Cajal famously said.

Cajal truly was a humanist and a polymath, in the Renaissance tradition. His legacy transcends brain science. Although the majority of his work concerns the nervous system, Cajal was a physician who contributed to many other fields. To pathology, he contributed studies on tuberculosis, leprosy, syphilis, rabies, and Alzheimer's disease.[45] His work on cancer is notable for the first description of an initial stage breast-cell carcinoma, and he seems to presage the idea of the stem cell.[46] Under his pseudonym "Doctor Bacteria," he also published findings on the vaccine for cholera, one year before its official discovery. In addition to monographs and journal articles, Cajal authored several editions of successful textbooks in an attempt to elevate science education in his native country. His *Manual of General Anatomical Pathology and Pathological Bacteriology* (1890) was updated for ten new editions during his lifetime.

In addition to his scientific work, Cajal also wrote books for a general audience. As his international fame grew, he became a public intellectual and a member of the renowned "Generation of '98," a group, including figures such as Miguel de Unamuno and Azorín, that wanted to rehabilitate the culture of Spain. He contributed articles on progressive education reform to a journal that also featured the bylines of Darwin, Tagore, Dewey, and a host of other luminaries; he penned forewords to contemporary books, one of which reveals his socialist ideology based on his interpretations of "natural" law; and he produced one of the earliest manuals on color photography in Spain. The titles of his newspaper articles suggest an eclecticism of interests, from pregnancy to wine and bees.

In the final quarter of his life, Cajal published *Café Chats*,[47] a collection of aphorisms and meditations inspired by *tertulias*, intellectual circles similar to Paris salons. His last book, *The World as Seen by an Eighty-Year-Old*,[48] is a painstaking account of his deterioration and decline. His more personal books were valuable enough to him that when he died, he explicitly instructed his students to read his autobiography, *Recollections of My Life*, and his scientific guide, *Advice for a Young Investigator*.[49] Along with many of his scientific classics, these two have been translated into English, as has his volume of science fiction, *Vacation Stories*, also as Doctor Bacteria.

The dream diary of Santiago Ramón y Cajal, only recently uncovered and never before read by Anglophones, offers a rare and intimate glimpse into the psyche of its legendary author.

REFERENCES

1. Pedro Calderón de la Barca, *Life Is a Dream*, trans. Gregary Racz (New York: Penguin Classics, 2006).
2. George Makari, *Revolution in Mind* (New York: Harper Perennial, 2009).
3. Abdellatif Nemri, "Santiago Ramón y Cajal," *Scholarpedia* 5, no. 12 (2010), 8577. doi:10.4249/scholarpedia.8577.
4. Santiago Ramón y Cajal, *Recollections of My Life*, trans. E. Horne Craigie with Juan Cano (Cambridge, Massachusetts: MIT Press, 1989), 363.
5. See Juan Fernández Rodríguez, "Cajal–Freud: Vidas cruzadas," *Revista de Psicoterapia y Psicosomática* 30, no.73 (2010), 9–12.
6. Casey Schwartz, *In the Mind Fields: Exploring the New Science of Neuropsychoanalysis* (Pantheon: New York, 2015); Allan Schore, "A Century After Freud's Project for Scientific Psychology: Is a Rapprochement Between Psychoanalysis and Neurobiology at Hand?" *Journal of the American Psychiatric Association* 45 (1997), 807–839.
7. Francisco López-Muñoz, Cecilio Alamo, and Gabriel Rubio, "The Neurobiological Interpretation of the Mental Functions in the Work of Santiago Ramón y Cajal," *History of Psychiatry* 19, no. 1 (2008), 18. doi:10.1177/0957X06075783.
8. Dorothy Cannon, *Explorer of the Human Brain* (New York: Schuman, 1949), 261.
9. José Rallo Romero, Francisco Martí Felipo and Miguel Ángel Jiménez-Arriero, *Los Sueños de santiago Ramón y Cajal* (Madrid: Biblioteca Nueva, 2014).
10. George Bush, "Decade of the Brain, 1990–1999, Proclamation 6158" (July 17, 1990).
11. "Brain Initiative" (September 30, 2014), https://www.whitehouse.gov/share/brain-initiative.
12. Nature Magazine, "Human Brain Project Needs a Rethink," *Scientific American* (March 14, 2015), http://www.scientificamerican.com/article/human-brain-project-needs-a-rethink.
13. For more criticism of this trend, see Amir Muzur and Iva Rinčić, "Neurocriticism: A Contribution to the Study of the Etiology, Phenomenology, and Ethics of the Use and Abuse of the Prefix Neuro-," *European Journal of Bioethics* 4, no. 7 (2013); Davi Johnston Thornton, *Brain Culture: Neuroscience and Popular Media* (New Brunswick, New Jersey: Rutgers University Press, 2011); "'Brain Culture': How Neuroscience Became a Pop Culture Fixation," *The Atlantic* (August 18, 2011), http://www.theatlantic.com/health/archive/2011/08/brain-culture-how-neuroscience-became-a-pop-culturefixation/243810; Steven Poole, "Your Brain on Pseudoscience: The Rise of Popular Neurobollocks," *New Statesman* (September 6, 2012), http://www.newstatesman.com/culture/books/2012/09/your-brain-pseudoscience-rise-popular-neurobollocks; Sally Satel and Scott O. Littlefield, *Brainwashed: The Seductive Appeal of Mindless Neuroscience* (New York: Basic Books, 2013).
14. José María López Piñero, *Santiago Ramón y Cajal* (Valencia: Universitat de València, 2006).
15. Evan Connell, *Aztec Treasure House: New and Selected Essays* (Berkeley, California: Counterpoint, 2002).
16. Plinio Prioreschi, "Possible Reasons for Neolithic Skull Trephining," *Perspectives in Biology and Medicine* 34, no. 2 (Winter 1991), 301.

17. Hippocrates, *On the Sacred Disease*, trans. Francis Adams, http://classics.mit.edu/Hippocrates/sacred.html.

18. Javier DeFelipe, "Sesquicentenary of the Birth of Santiago Ramón y Cajal," *Trends in Neuroscience* 25, no. 9 (2002), 484. doi:10.1016/S01666-2236(02)02214-2; Frank W. Stahnisch and Robert Nitsch, "Santiago Ramón y Cajal's Concept of Neuronal Plasticity: The Ambiguity Lives On," *Trends in Neurosciences* 25, no. 11 (2002), 589. doi:10.1016/S0166-2236(02)02251-8.

19. L. W. Swanson, "Preface to the American Translation," in *The Histology of the Nervous System*, trans. Neely Swanson and Larry Swanson (New York: Oxford University Press, 1991), xxi.

20. Gordon Shepherd, *The Foundation of the Neuron Doctrine* (New York: Oxford University Press, 1991), 127.

21. Charles Sherrington, "A Memoir to Dr. Cajal," introduction to *Explorer of the Human Brain*, by Dorothy Cannon (New York: Schuman, 1949), xii.

22. Marina Bentivoglio and Paolo Mazzarello, "The Anatomical Foundations of Clinical Neurology," in *History of Neurology*, ed. Stanley Finger, François Boller, and Kenneth L. Tyler; *Handbook of Clinical Neurology* vol. 95, ed. Michael J. Aminoff, François Boller, and Dick F. Swaab (Amsterdam: Elsevier, 2010), 163.

23. Swanson, "Preface," *Histology*, xxvii.

24. "Santiago Ramón y Cajal," Google Scholar Citations, https://scholar.google.es/citations?user=K3LMrNIAAAAJ&hl=en (accessed May 1, 2016).

25. "Brief History," *History of the Cajal Club*," http://cajalclub.org/id3.html, and a private conversation with a club member.

26. "Homage to Cajal [Tattoo]," at "The Loom, a Blog by Carl Zimmer," at *Phenomenon: A Science Salon* (January 20, 2009), http://phenomena.nationalgeographic.com/2009/01/20/1472.

27. "You can be for ccajal or against him but not without him!" writes Marcus Jacobson in *The Foundations of Neuroscience* (New York: Plenum Press, 1995), 233.

28. Miguel A. Merchán, Javier DeFelipe, and Fernando de Castro, *Cajal and De Castro's Neurohistological Methods* (New York: Oxford University Press, 2016), 14.

29. The Asturias miners strike.

30. Santiago Ramón y Cajal, *Café Chats*, 5th edition (Buenos Aires: Espasa Calpe, 1948).

31. Javier DeFelipe, *Cajal's Butterflies of the Soul: Science and Art* (New York: Oxford University Press, 2009), 3.

32. DeFelipe, *Butterflies of the Soul*, 29.

33. Sidney Ochs, *A History of Nerve Function: From Animal Spirits to Molecular Mechanisms* (Cambridge, UK: Cambridge University Press, 2004), 1–2.

34. Cajal, *Recollections*, 252.

35. Cajal, *Recollections*, 278.

36. Santiago Ramón y Cajal (Doctor Bacteria). "Las maravillas de la Histología," *La Clínica* 301, 303, 304, 305, 310, 312, 313 (1883): 225–226; 241–242; 249–250; 257–258; 297–299; 313–315, 321–323.

37. Cajal, *Recollections*, 131.

38. Cajal, *Recollections*, 373.

39. Sherrington, "A Memoir to Dr. Cajal" in *Explorer of the Human Brain*, xiii–xiv.

40. Sherrington, "A Memoir to Dr. Cajal," xiv.

41. *Cajal's Degeneration and Regeneration of the Nervous System*, trans. Raoul M. May (New York: Oxford University Press, 1991).

42. Santiago Ramón y Cajal, *Neuron Theory or Reticular Theory? Objective Evidence of the Anatomical Unity of Nerve Cells*, trans. M. Ubeda Purkiss and Clement A. Fox

(Madrid: Consejo Superior de Investigaciones Científicas, Instituto Ramón y Cajal, 1951).

43. On Cajal's aesthetic practices, see Sarah de Rijcke, "Drawing into Abstraction: Practices of Observation and Visualization in the Work of Santiago Ramón y Cajal," *Interdisciplinary Science Reviews* 33, no. 4 (December 2008), 287–311. doi:10.11.79/174327908X392861; Erna Fiorentini, "Inducing Visibilities: An Attempt at Santiago Ramón y Cajal's Aesthetic Epistemology," *Studies in History and Philosophy Part C: Studies in History and Philosopher of Biological and Biomedical Sciences* 42, no. 4 (December 2011), 391–394; Pablo Garcia-López, Virginia Garcia-Marín, and Miguel Freire, "The Histological Slides and Drawings of Cajal," *Frontiers in Neuroanatomy* 4 (March 10, 2010). doi:10.3389/neuro.05.009.2010; and DeFelipe, *Cajal's Butterflies of the Soul.*

44. *Fisiología de los sueños: Cajal, Tanguy, Lorca, Dali* ... (Catálogos Paranínfo); "Architecture of Life," at the University of California–Berkeley Art Museum and Pacific Film Archive, in Berkeley, California; "States of Mind: Tracing the Edges of Consciousness," at the Wellcome Collection in London, England.

45. Nemri, "Santiago Ramón y Cajal."

46. A. Martinez, "The Contributions of Santiago Ramón y Cajal to Cancer Research—100 Years On," *Nature Reviews Cancer* 5 (November 2005), 904–909.

47. Santiago Ramón y Cajal, *Charlas de café: Pensamientos, anécdotas y confidencias* (Madrid: Juan Pueyo, 1921).

48. Santiago Ramón y Cajal, *El mundo visto a los ochenta años: Impresiones de un arteriosclerótico*, 5th edition (Buenos Aires: Espasa-Calpe, 1948).

49. Santiago Ramón y Cajal, *Advice for a Young Investigator*, trans. Neely Swanson and Larry W. Swanson (Cambridge, Massachusetts: MIT Press, 1999).

CHAPTER 2

⌐∿⌐

Cajal and Psychology

In the second half of the nineteenth century, psychological inquiry shifted away from the realm of philosophy and into the natural sciences, revolutionizing the study of the human mind.[1] In the past, the inner world of human beings had seemed utterly inaccessible. How could the self be an object of rational inquiry? On the other hand, the associationalist school, founded by British empiricists, believed that the basic elements of the psyche were thoughts, feelings, sensations, and perceptions, which were available to study. Associationalist psychology investigated the causes and effects among these impressions and looked at the human mind as a mechanical loom that weaves together separate strands of mental experience into a unified pattern of consciousness.[2] For scientists of the mind, this was a promising model that encouraged investigators such as Cajal to search for the anatomical basis of the mind. "To know the brain," Cajal thought at the time, "is equivalent to ascertaining the material course of thought and will."[3] In order to be rational and objective, psychology including the study of dreaming, would have to correspond to the anatomy of the brain.

Cajal's discovery of distinctly individual cells inside the brain seemed to confirm the associationalist model. Neurons were the units of the mind, each able to store an impression, an appealing schema of one-to-one correspondence. In the 1890s, Cajal was reading and engaging with the ideas of prominent associationalist thinkers such as Ivan Petrovich Pavlov and William James.[4] In the company of the great psychologists of his day, he theorized about the cellular bases of consciousness, memory, and attention, and although his contributions to this field are fewer and not as well known, his insights as a psychologist deserve our attention.

Of the three hundred and fifty scientific articles published by Cajal, only eight—or two percent—are oriented explicitly toward the subject of psychology. Counting prefaces to popular books, speeches, and editions, the psychological ouevre of Cajal is composed of a total of twelve titles. This number is both extremely low, compared to the great European psychologists, and relatively high, compared to his peers in Spain.[5] Cajal's attitude toward psychological research reflects a characteristic pattern of his scientific thinking: Beginning as close to the "purest ideal of neurohistology"[6] as possible, he experimented with physiological interpretations of the anatomical facts as foundational material for a potential empirical theory, until finally he was forced to confront the inability of this reductionist method to explain the more complex emergent phenomena of mind. This intellectual habit, which contributed to his discipline as a scientific researcher, also determined how he treated his forays into more tempting popular research topics, such as dreaming.

In a 1892 lecture, later published as *The New Concept of the Histology of the Nervous System*,[7] Cajal tackles the cellular bases of higher mental function with trademark rigor and aplomb. The common belief within the scientific community at the time was that the human brain and the brains of other mammals differed on account of our greater *quantity* of cells. Alternatively, Cajal wondered whether "the psychological nobility of *Homo sapiens*" was due to a *qualitative* and not *quantitative* difference between the brains of human beings and other mammals. Like all material composition, the form of the neuron must constrain the function of the nervous system, according to the laws of nature. Therefore, he set out "to reveal these enigmatic, strictly human neurons upon which our zoological superiority is founded." Most localists at the time, including Cajal, homed in on the most recently evolved area in the brain—the cerebral cortex—as the potential seat of our most sophisticated capabilities. In the cerebral cortex, Cajal discovered that a distinctive type of cell, "the pyramidal cell," is absent in lower mammals, becomes larger and more complex as one ascends the animal scale, and is abundantly rich in human beings. "It is natural," he concludes, "to attribute this progressive morphological complexity, in part at least, to its progressive functional state." He inferred that these spindly, fragile-looking cells are the units of psychological function, and he dubbed them "the psychic cells."[8]

In May 1894, Cajal elaborated on his ideas about the psychic cell in the prestigious Croonian Lecture at the Royal Academy of Science in London.[9] Having observed that the protoplasmic processes, the nineteenth-century term for *dendrites*, were more greatly differentiated and abundant in psychic cells, whereas the collateral and terminal nervous branches, the nineteenth-century term for *axons*, were more numerous, he inferred that the psychic cell must have developed a more complex morphology in order to carry out a more complex function. He found that more primitive animals do not have large psychic cells and that the connections from these cells to others are local; higher animals, on the other hand, have *thousands* of connections that extend *far* into different regions, even all the way down to the spinal cord. Cajal proposed that this elaborate connectivity of cells enhanced the ability of these cells to function within integrative circuits, allowing them to combine impressions and synthesize images. This lent concrete grounding to the associationalist vision: one-to-one correspondence between the unit of impression and the cell, and the potential for these cells to pattern connections among themselves to an exponential order of permutations high enough that the output of the machine might approach a casual explanation of the unfathomable complexity of conscious experience.

At his most speculative, Cajal stretches his interpretation of the neuron theory to an almost mystical realm. In 1896, he published *Interpretaciones conjeturales sobre algunos puntos de histo-fisiología neurológica*,[10] or *Conjectural Interpretations on Some Points of Neurological Physiology*, in which he stretches the neuron theory further. If the cell is the unit of psychology, for storage of mental impressions, then the nervous system would consist of innumerable consciousnesses, "as many as there are cells, with a cerebral one, superior, and with autocracy over all the rest."[11] This granular hierarchy hints at Cajal's concept of the psyche, upon which he would elaborate later in his life. "What we would call the *self*, or the person," he continues, "would be none other than the cerebral consciousness, which is ignorant of—as it is exterior to—the conscious *self* of all the subordinate ganglionic individualities."[12] The accessibility of the self and relationship among our internal formations are subjects to which Cajal alludes in a particularly confounding entry in the dream diary. These ideas echo the tone and perspective of Cajal's earlier more philosophical essays, printed in local medical journals with the byline Dr. Bacteria.[13] The anonymity of this pseudonym allowed him to express himself at the fringes of scientific thought, although later, in the fullness of his maturity, he disavowed these flights of imagination, judging his alter ego as "dreadful."

Cajal believed that scientific discovery required many intellectual traits in harmonious combination. He tempered his idealism with "a sound critical judgment that is able to reject the rash impulses of daydreams in favor of those thoughts most faithfully embracing objective reality."[14] In 1897, Cajal planned to deliver a speech to the Royal Academy of Medicine in Spain, which he titled, "The Physiologic–Psychological Inductions Deriving from Recent Histological Research." In the end, he did not deliver that speech because he judged the research as "incomplete and premature."[15] Instead, he made a safer choice, removing the physiologic–psychological inductions and speaking strictly in terms of histology. The first Spanish edition of *The Texture of the Nervous System*, released in 1899, included a section on the origins of thought, will, and consciousness, which he then redacted in subsequent editions. Cajal called himself "a fervent adept of the religion of facts," whose dogma was that "hypotheses come and go but facts remain."[16]

In the final analysis, Cajal was skeptical about the associationalist quest for a scientific psychology. He stated in his Croonian Lecture speech,

> As things stand today, it cannot be denied that objective psychology or mental histology [two names for the aforementioned task] is a nascent science, whose purpose is to subordinate the series of mental acts reflected in consciousness to a parallel series of physico-mental phenomena affected by cells, is still largely reduced to the quite primitive and speculative method of the physiological interpretation of the anatomical evidence.[17]

His notebooks from earlier in his career, before his breakthrough discoveries, reveal the sketch of a humorous science fiction story, posthumously released, that treats this theme. *Life in the Year 6000* is about a nineteenth-century doctor who is reanimated in the distant future, where another doctor explains the changes in the world to him. The imaginary doctor reflects on the "ancient" tendency—from Cajal's own era—toward immaterial theorizing, which he calls a "cerebral deformity."[18] Primitive and speculative methods never satisfied him. Although he had faith in the resources of the human brain, Cajal knew that contemporary neuroanatomy was incapable of explaining psychology. "All the most intimate and crucial aspects of mental life," he writes, "stay in the background."[19] Dreaming was among the cast of dimly understood phenomena that Cajal tried to examine on center stage.

REFERENCES

1. George Makari, Revolution in Mind (New York: Harper Perennial, 2008).
2. Makari, *Revolution in Mind*, 10–14.
3. Cajal, *Recollections*, 305.
4. Maria Dolores Saiz and Milgaros Saiz, *Personajes para una historia de la psicología en españa* (Madrid: Piramide, 1995), 205.
5. López-Muñoz et al., "The Neurobiological Interpretation of the Mental Functions in the Work of Santiago Ramón y Cajal," 7.
6. de Rijcke, "Drawing into Abstraction," 306.
7. López-Muñoz et al., "The Neurobiological Interpretation of the Mental Functions in the Work of Santiago Ramón y Cajal."

8. Patricia Goldman-Rakic, "The 'Psychic Cell' of Ramón y Cajal," *Progress in Brain Research* 136 (2002), 427–434.

9. Edward G. Jones, "Santiago Ramón y Cajal and the Croonian Lecture, March 1894," *Trends in Neurosciences* 17, no. 5 (1994), 190–192.

10. Santiago Ramón y Cajal, "Interpretaciones conjeturales sobre algunos puntos de histo-fisiología neurológica," *Biblioteca de la Ciencia Moderna*, 379–392.

11. López-Muñoz et al., "The Neurobiological Interpretation of the Mental Functions in the Work of Santiago Ramón y Cajal."

12. López-Muñoz, et al., "The Neurobiological Interpretation of the Mental Functions in the Work of Santiago Ramón y Cajal."

13. See Cajal, "Los actos reflejos y la filosofía del inconsciente," *La Clínica* (1881) and "Las maravillas de la Histología," *La Clínica* (1883).

14. Cajal, *Advice*, 29.

15. López-Muñoz et al., "The Neurobiological Interpretation of the Mental Functions in the Work of Santiago Ramón y Cajal," 14.

16. Cajal, *Recollections*, 455; Cajal, *Advice*, 86.

17. López-Muñoz et al., "The Neurobiological Interpretations of the Mental Functions in the Work of Santiago Ramón y Cajal," 11.

18. *La vida en el año 6000: Biblioteca Ramón y Cajal autografos de Cajal*, ed. García Durán Muñoz and Nana Ramón y Cajal de Durán (Cáceres, Spain: Tip. Extremadura, 1973), 10.

19. López-Muñoz et al., "The Neurobiological Interpretations of the Mental Functions in the Work of Santiago Ramón y Cajal," 15.

CHAPTER 3

꧁

Cajal and Dream Research

Although the history of dream research is storied and ancient, scientific investigations into dreaming officially began in the nineteenth century.[1] In 1855, the philosophy section of the French publication *Academie des Sciences Morales et Politiques* proposed a competition for theories of sleep and dreams from a psychological perspective.[2] Both professional scientists and laypeople participated. Guiding questions were "What mental faculties subsist, or stop, or change considerably during sleep?" and "What is the fundamental difference between dreaming and thinking?" At the time, most dream researchers believed that dreams were exclusively caused by external stimulation, and their investigations were phenomenological in concern.[3] For example, Alfred Maury challenged the idea of dreams as supernatural in origin by recording the effects of physical impressions, such as a feather tickling his face, on thousands of his dreams.[4] Another influential researcher, Hervey de Saint-Denis, who continuously recorded his dreams for five years, would douse his servants' pillows with perfume without telling them and note changes in their dreams the next morning.[5] Positivists tended to view dream content as the meaningless by-product of random brain activity and did not engage in interpretation. Artists and writers in the Romantic movement were among the cultural figures fascinated by dreaming;[6] perhaps the most relevant example of their interest is an etching by Francisco José de Goya y Lucientes, an Aragonese Spaniard like Cajal, called "The Sleep of Reason Produces Monsters."

In a 1902 preface to a contemporary poetry book, Cajal makes a similar statement, which he tries to prove with a theory involving cells. In an attempt to illuminate how the brain can alternate between modes of comedy and drama, Cajal explains that some cells are active during our daily routine, whereas others are unproductive, as though lying in a fallow field. These idle cells, alienated by their unemployment, will "loudly demand a turn at the banquet." In Cajal's characteristically anthropomorphic view, the agency is theirs; they increase their blood flow, they activate themselves, and their different and unconventional contributions are what lead to our creative thinking. Cajal writes,

> Everyone will have noticed that when we sleep, the ideas and events in the special world that unfolds before us are usually (and there are exceptions that if we think about it actually prove the rule) totally unconnected with the thoughts that preoccupy us and with our everyday tasks and demands.

Natural lulls in our brain activity occur during sleep, and so this is when protests of these previously dormant cells are most successful. Dreams, then, are akin to a rebellion by our brain cells.

Cajal writes,

> If we analyze dreams carefully, we see that they often involve scenes from our childhood or youth, rarely remembered, or capriciously fragmented and absurdly combined images, whose sensory elements and residues have not been refreshed for a long time, so that they remain outside the field of consciousness.

He calls this unconscious "a kind of reserve of ideas." "When we sleep," he writes, "we do not rest completely . . . the cells in which unconscious images are recorded stay awake and become excited, rejuvenating themselves with the exercise they did behind the back of the conscious mind." The cells throughout the brain that are hyperactive during daytime operations—especially those responsible for "the critical faculty"—are exhausted and rest; meanwhile, the fresh cells that store unused impressions are free to perform their gymnastics, randomly synthesizing their impulses. "The majority of dreams," Cajal concludes, "consists of scraps of ideas, unconnected or weirdly assembled, somewhat like an absurd monster without proportions, harmony, or reason."[7]

Cajal published only one scientific paper on dreaming.[8] Although he did not value the content of dreams, he was fascinated by their neurobiological mechanisms. "Dreaming is one of the most interesting and most wondrous physiological phenomena in the brain," Cajal writes to begin his 1908 article "Theories of Dreaming."[9] Cajal was curious about the mechanisms behind visual hallucination and perception in dreams. To study these questions, he conducted thousands of self-explorations. His method was to utilize autosuggestion the day before sleep, training himself to have visual dreams by creation of habit, which he called "the introspective method." Although he reports that the method worked only once or twice out of a hundred times, he believed that the practice eventually would lead to better results. Cajal did have enough success to report some material, such as dreams in which he finds himself in the middle of a dense forest, walks on the street in Madrid, and examines a book. He does not bother to interpret them; rather, he uses them as experimental data to investigate the color, perspective, and relief of dream imagery as well as the physiology of visual dreaming.[10]

True to form, Cajal's focus is on the anatomical substrate beneath the mental phenomena. He wanted to know *where* in the brain the physiological activity that causes dreams is happening, a focus known as "localist."[11] "Do they arise in the associative, higher or project centers?" he asks about visions in dreams. "Are the retina and the optic nerve involved?" Through analysis of thousands of dreams, he concluded that there was no involvement from any cells in the retina. His definitive evidence was from experiments with "people who went blind as adults; those who could populate their memory in the early years of their life with pictures dream with optical images, despite lacking both retina and optic nerve." In other words, with no peripheral stimulation, these subjects still experienced visual dreaming, which meant that dreams were internal constructions. Cajal's only article on dreaming ends promisingly, with the words "To be continued. . . ."[12] For a decade, however, he did not. Given that dream research existed at his scientific margins, this delay is to be expected. The question is not why he immediately did not continue but, rather, why he resumed at all.

REFERENCES

1. Sophie Schwartz, "A Historical Loop of 100 Years: Similarities Between 19th Century and Contemporary Dream Research," *Dreaming* 10, no. 1 (2000), 55–66. doi:10.1023/a:1009455807975.
2. Schwartz, "A Historical Loop of 100 Years: Similarities Between 19th Century and Contemporary Dream Research," 56.
3. Schwartz, "A Historical Loop of 100 Years: Similarities Between 19th Century and Contemporary Dream Research," 56.
4. J. Allan Hobson, *The Dreaming Brain* (New York: Basic Books, 1988), 33–34.
5. Hobson, *The Dreaming Brain*, 33–34.
6. Laura Marcus, "Introduction: Histories, Representations, Autobiographics in *The Interpretation of Dreams*," in *The Interpretation of Dreams: New Interdisciplinary Essays*, ed. Laura Marcus (Manchester, UK: Manchester University Press, 1999), 13.
7. All quotations from Cajal's 1902 "Preface" are taken from Lazaros C. Triarhou and Ana B. Rivas, "Poetry and the Brain: Cajal's Conjectures on the Psychology of Writers,"

Perspectives in Biology and Medicine 52, no. 1 (Winter 2009), 80–89. doi:10.1353/pbm.0.0069; López-Muñoz et al., "The Neurobiological Interpretation of the Mental Functions in the Work of Santiago Ramón y Cajal."

8. López-Muñoz et al., "The Neurobiological Interpretation of the Mental Functions in the Work of Santiago Ramón y Cajal," 9.

9. For excerpts from Cajal's 1908 "Theories of Dreaming," see López-Muñoz et al., "The Neurobiological Interpretation of the Mental Functions in the Work of Santiago Ramón y Cajal."

10. López-Muñoz et al., "The Neurobiological Interpretation of the Mental Functions in the Work of Santiago Ramón y Cajal, 19."

11. Maria Nazarova and Evgeny Blagovechtchenski, "Modern Brain Mapping— What Do We Map Nowadays?" *Frontiers in Psychiatry* 6 (2015), 89. doi:10.3389/fpsyt.2015.00089.

12. López-Muñoz et al., "The Neurobiological Interpretations of the Mental Functions in the Work of Santiago Ramón y Cajal," 17.

CHAPTER 4

ᐧᐤᐧ

Cajal and Freudianism in Spain

Do you suppose that some day a marble tablet with be placed on the house, inscribed with the words: "In this house on July 24, 1895, the Secret of Dreams was revealed to Dr. Sigmund Freud"? At this moment I see little prospect of it.[1]

Sigmund Freud, letter to Wilhelm Fleiss (1900)

When Sigmund Freud released his dream book, *Die Traumdeutung*, in 1900, the world initially failed to notice. For a year and a half, no scientific journal reviewed the book and only few periodicals mentioned it.[2] Less than four hundred copies were sold in the first six years after publication; the initial printing of six hundred copies did not sell through for eight years. "Oh, how glad I am that no one knows . . .," Freud wrote in a letter. "No one even suspects that the dream is not nonsense but wish-fulfillment."[3] In *The Interpretation of Dreams*, Freud claims to have a physiological technique that allows him to interpret the meaning of dreams. According to Freud, dreams have dual layers; the *manifest content*, apparent to the dreamer, reflects the symbolic expression of *latent content*, the true hidden meaning. Scandalously, he proposed that sexual desires experienced since infancy are present unconsciously in the adult psyche. A censor in the mind normally acts to repress this and other unconscious material, which then is released in the form of dreams.[4] Freud's dream theories were central to his doctrine of psychoanalysis; the interpretation of dreams became a method for psychiatric treatment, helping patients to resolve their internal conflicts and relieving their burdensome emotions.

Spain was among the countries most receptive to Freud and psychoanalysis.[5] In 1893, the first foreign translation of Freud, excerpts from his book on hysteria, was published in a relatively obscure Spanish

(23)

journal, surprising even Freud. When Freud first developed his theories, only German speakers were able to access his writings. Those people, mostly doctors and other academics, often gathered to discuss the more salacious ideas. Then, in 1911, the philosopher José Ortega y Gasset, who studied German in the city of Marburg, published an article titled "Psychoanalysis: A Problematic Science," including a section titled "The Secret of Dreams." Although skeptical of some aspects of Freudian theory, the essay effectively popularized Freud in Spain. Cajal must have read this; even if he had encountered Freud's theories previously, this publication signified a new degree of prominence. "At heart," Ortega summarizes, "Freud is trying to make psychophysiology lead into biology, and I find nothing to oppose in this tendency."[6] In contrast, at heart, Cajal was trying to make biology lead into psychophysiology. The two neurologists were moving toward the same aim from opposite directions.

After a decade of research with a new histological stain, in 1913, Cajal published another monumental work, *Degeneration and Regeneration of the Nervous System*. His research during that period addressed the most pressing questions of contemporary neuroanatomy: How do neurons recover from damage and what kind of damage can they recover from? Can neurons always repair themselves, or is there an age after which this potential no longer exists? Is there any kind of damage that would be considered beyond repair?[7] In 1914, Cajal, along with his students, was scheduled to attend a neuroscience conference in Zurich and present new findings. This was to be an auspicious moment for the Spanish school of neurobiology, which Cajal founded. Since the beginning of his career, Cajal's stated mission was to elevate the homegrown culture of Spanish science to the level of that in other European countries. Tragically, this was the year that Archduke Franz Ferdinand was assassinated, triggering the outbreak of World War I. The Zurich conference was canceled, and Cajal was unable to communicate with any of his colleagues.[8] Cajal's isolation from the scientific world coincided with the formal introduction of psychoanalysis to the medical discourse in Spain, when a 1914 Spanish book on hysteria appeared with a chapter on psychoanalysis.[9]

Psychoanalysis was the subject of much debate among the intellectual life in Madrid. Every day, Cajal participated in *tertulias* with his familiar circle at their favorite café, and he often attended the Atheneum, a private cultural center, where he met other prominent colleagues and friends, including Ortega.[10] These conversations must have included Freud's provocative ideas. Despite their political differences, both liberals and conservatives were known to embrace psychoanalysis. Even those who rejected Freud's ideas served to amplify his message with the vehemence of their public antagonism. The popularity of Freud in his home country surprised and confused Cajal.[11] As the only Spanish scientist to win a Nobel Prize, he occupied a position of intellectual authority, which he coveted. Much to his dismay and frustration, his fellow Spaniards were glorifying a foreigner while the world was ignoring him. In 1917, Ortega convinced a Spanish editor to contact Freud and acquire the rights to his complete works, the first in any language. Although Spain was technically neutral, negotiations were precarious, conducted through the Spanish embassy in Vienna, with copies of Freud's works shuttled across battlefront countries in diplomatic pouches.[12]

In this intellectual climate, even Cajal's own students started warming to Freud. Leading the charge, two of Cajal's closest disciples, Gonzalo Lafora and José M. Sacristán, published articles on psychoanalysis in *El Sol*,[13] the liberal newspaper with which Ortega was affiliated, which Cajal certainly would have read.[14] Although rejecting Freud's theories of sexuality, their articles demonstrate that the next generation of Spanish scientists had come to accept many of his views, including "the reality of repressed complexes and their symbolic exteriorization in dreams."[15] Despite Cajal's more absolutist doctrine, his students were willing to reconcile psychoanalysis with traditional biology, seizing on the more positivistic and evolutionary elements of the theory. In the aftermath of Einsteinian relativity, this younger cohort was far more comfortable with the role of subjectivity in science[16] than Cajal, devotee of objective fact.[17] In Cajal's mind, not only was Freud a foreigner; he was also a heretic.

"There are two phases in a man's life," writes the Spanish journalist Wenceslao Fernández Flórez, "before reading Freud and after."[18] In the first phase of Cajal's life, he expressed his belief that dreams are meaningless and published scientific research on dreaming as a visual phenomenon. Cajal embarked on his dream project in the "second phase," after Freud's ideas had penetrated Spain. From the first entry of the diary, Cajal's purpose is clear: He intends to test Freud's theories against the observations of his own dreams. Cajal summarized the basic concept of dreams as fulfillments of repressed desire and more vaguely refers to other ideas, such as infantile sexuality ("sexual in origin"), symbolism ("something else appears"), the day's residue ("the evocative cause"), and the role of the internal censor ("the lack of reason").[19] Cajal may have claimed that dreams were meaningless, but their lack of meaning suddenly seemed deeply meaningful to him.

In 1922, the first volume of the *Collected Works of Sigmund Freud*, a Spanish translation of *The Psychopathology of Everyday Life*, was released. Freud complimented the translator, Luis López Ballesteros, "for the most correct interpretation of my thought and the elegance of style."[20] The series was an immediate commercial success; it seemed that every intellectual and professional in Madrid bought a volume. *The Psychopathology of Everyday Life* and *The Interpretation of Dreams*, the most popular install-ments of the series,[21] were among the books in Cajal's personal library.[22] His reading habit was to scribble comments in the margins of books, as though in conversation with their authors.[23] "The interpretation is so subtle (in the forgetting of verses, words and phrases)," one page of Freud reads, "that it is impossible to believe the author."[24] "It seems strange," Cajal writes toward the end of his life, "that such a keen and encyclopedic intellect should commit such grave errors."[25]

According to Gregorio Marañon, the famous medical scientist and writer who was Cajal's friend, former student, and the only Spanish doc-tor to meet Freud, Cajal was never enthusiastic but always respectful, even calling him "the wise Viennese professor."[26] However, his animosity is revealed in private letters. "I consider as collective lies both psychoanaly-sis and Freud's theory of dreams," he writes, "Of this I shall manage to live long enough to write another book on dreams." He writes in another let-ter, "In more than five hundred dreams I have analyzed (without counting those of the people I know), it is impossible to verify, except in extremely rare cases, the doctrines of the surly and somewhat egotistical Viennese author."[27] In 1928, Sándor Ferenczi, a Hungarian psychoanalyst and close associate of Freud for a time, traveled to Spain and delivered a lecture, but Cajal chose not to attend, even though many of his colleagues did so. Instead, Cajal was engaged in an imaginary conversation with Freud, in the dream diary he faithfully composed.

REFERENCES

1. "1895: Sigmund Freud Chronology," *Sigmund Freud Museum Vienna*, http://www.freud-museum.at/online/freud/chronolg/1895-e.htm.
2. "Freud's Book, 'The Interpretation of Dreams,' Released 1900," *A Science Odyssey: Peoples and Discoveries* (PBS), http://www.pbs.org/wgbh/aso/databank/entries/dh00fr.html.
3. Anne-Marie Rizzuto, *Why Did Freud Reject God? A Psychodynamic Interpretation* (New Haven, Connecticut: Yale University Press, 1998), 84.
4. "Freud's book," PBS.org.
5. Thomas Glick, "The Naked Science: Psychoanalysis in Spain, 1914–1948," *Comparative Studies in Society and History* 24, no. 4 (1982), 533–571, http://isites.harvard.edu/fs/docs/icb.topic355408.files/Freud/Freud_Spain.pdf.
6. Glick, "The Naked Science," 540.
7. R. D. Lobato, "Historical Vignette of Cajal's Work 'Degeneration and Regeneration of the Nervous System' with a Reflection by the Author," *Neurocirugía* 19 (2008), 456–468, http://scielo.isciii.es/pdf/neuro/v19n5/8.pdf.
8. López Piñero, *Santiago Ramón y Cajal*, 333–353.
9. Glick, "The Naked Science," 537.

10. Rallo et al., *Los sueños*, 75–77.
11. Rallo et al., *Los sueños*, 75–77.
12. Glick, "The Naked Science," 540.
13. Glick, "The Naked Science," 538
14. Glick, "The Naked Science," 248.
15. Glick, "The Naked Science," 538.
16. Glick, "The Naked Science."
17. Cajal, *Recollections*, 455.
18. Cajal, *Recollections*, 533.
19. First entry of the dream diary, as translated in the present book (Ehrlich, *The Dreams of Santiago Ramón y Cajal*).
20. Glick, "The Naked Science," 541.
21. Glick, "The Naked Science," 540.
22. Jordi Rusiñol Estragués and Virgili Ibarz Serrat, "La recepción del pensamiento de Freud en la obra de Ramón y Cajal," *Persona* 6 (2003), 76.
23. Rusiñol Estragués and Ibarz Serrat, "La recepción del pensamiento de Freud en la obra de Ramón y Cajal," 76.
24. López-Muñoz et al., "The Neurobiological Interpretation of the Mental Functions in the Work of Santiago Ramón y Cajal," 18.
25. Rallo et al., *Los sueños*, 51.
26. Rallo et al., *Los sueños*, 24.
27. Rallo et al., *Los sueños*, 25.

CHAPTER 5

༽᠙ఌ

Comparing the Lives
of Cajal and Freud

Despite their many social and cultural differences, Santiago Ramón y Cajal and Sigmund Freud had more in common than one might naturally assume. Both grew up as provincial outsiders. Siegismund Schlomo Freud was born in the village of Freiburg in Moravia, an independent state on historical Czech land. His family was Jewish, a small and persecuted minority. Santiago Felipe Ramón y Cajal was born in the village of Petilla, isolated in the mountains of northern Spain. As children, Freud and Cajal were both precocious writers and readers. Whereas Freud had prodigious verbal gifts and was able to recite sophisticated academic texts from memory, Cajal was a visual learner who struggled with memorization but possessed natural artistic talent. Both Freud and Cajal idealized figures from literature and history and aspired to heroic achievement. For different reasons, both men became doctors. Neither intended to practice clinical medicine; Freud eventually capitulated, whereas Cajal never did. Both worked as anatomists and histologists of the nervous system while also experimenting with parapsychology, specifically hypnosis. Ultimately, the shared goal of "the father of modern neuroscience" and "the father of psychoanalysis" was to understand the human mind.[1] Despite developing within the same intellectual zeitgeist, their methods and visions dramatically diverged. The most fruitful exploration of this separation is through a brief comparison of their professional biographies.

In 1873, Cajal graduated with his surgical license from the University of Zaragoza medical school. His grades were average, except for anatomy and pathology, in which he excelled. Cajal was expected to earn his doctorate in medicine, the first step toward an academic career. However, when a Spanish conservative party rebelled against the liberal government, Cajal was drafted into the army, serving as a physician. Soon thereafter, wealthy plantation owners in the Spanish colony of Cuba seized the opportunity to declare their independence. At the height of the revolution, Cajal was sent to Cuba and promoted to captain. Stationed deep in the tropical jungle, he was in charge of a hospital, caring for hundreds of soldiers stricken with malaria and dysentery. "I lived as in a dream," Cajal would later recall of his time in Cuba, "and as if in a sort of spell."[2] The conditions were nightmarish; forced to sleep in the same room as the other soldiers, he soon contracted both diseases. Had he died then, like many of his comrades, no one would have ever known his name.

In the same year that Cajal entered into the army, Freud started his first term at the University of Vienna. Although he had many talents and interests, he decided to study medicine. His advisor was Ernst Brücke, a doctrinaire physiologist who swore an oath that "no other forces other than the common physical–chemical ones are active within the organism."[3] At the University of Vienna, Brücke established the first physiology institute in order to study the biological structure of the mind. Freud would write later that Brücke was "the greatest authority who affected me more than any other in my whole life."[4] Starting in 1877, Freud's mentor employed him as an anatomist in his laboratory. There, Freud practiced histology, dissecting tissues, staining them with chemicals, and examining them under the microscope to reveal their hidden architecture.

In Brücke's laboratory, Freud studied the lobes, spines, and organs of lamprey and crayfish. He investigated their nervous systems, comparing the anatomy of lower vertebrates to that of human beings. Freud demonstrated the evolution of sensory cells in human fibers from spinal cord cells in primitive fish.[5] His patient and ingenious technique, inspired by the theories of Darwin, was the same approach that Cajal would employ in his studies of the psychic cell. Like all histologists of his time, Freud had to draw what he saw on his slides in order to disseminate his findings. Although Cajal is the most famous artist of the brain, Freud's histological drawings of the nervous system found earlier success. His work appeared in the *Proceedings of the Imperial Academy of Sciences* a decade before Cajal even started to investigate the nervous system.[6] In the course of seven years in Brücke's laboratory, Freud published fourteen scientific articles on histology, neuroanatomy, and neuropathology. Moreover, he was happy. "In Ernst Brücke's laboratory," he writes, "I found rest and satisfaction."[7]

While Freud was excelling in histological research, a debilitated Cajal was convalescing at his parents' home in Zaragoza. When he recovered sufficiently, he took a job at his alma mater as an auxiliary professor of anatomy and as an assistant in the anatomical museum. He had yet to discover histology. The pivotal moment in his career came in 1878, when Cajal traveled to Madrid to study for his doctorate. There, he visited the laboratory of Maestre San Juan, a leading figure in Spanish anatomy, who showed Cajal how to prepare histological samples of organic tissue. Utterly amazed and inspired, Cajal decided to set up his own laboratory. At a time when microscopes were relatively uncommon in Spain—none of his colleagues in the university anatomy department used one—he arranged to purchase a cheaper instrument with his military back pay. Back in Zaragoza, a friend in the physiology laboratory with access to one of the rare models let him observe the circulation of blood in the gut of a frog through a microscope. Cajal was transfixed. "It was like a veil was lifted before my eyes," he later wrote, "There was presented to me a marvelous field for exploration, full of the most delightful surprises." Alone in his parents' cramped attic, Cajal began to explore new worlds, observing what he called "scenes in the life of the infinitely small."[8]

However, the demands of everyday life loomed large, standing in the way of his microscopic explorations. In Spain, lifetime academic appointments were determined by competitive examinations called *oposiciones*, judged by a bureaucratic tribunals not above political bias. For many reasons, Cajal failed; the trauma of oposiciones would haunt him for decades, as evidenced in his dreams. Still suffering the effects of his past illness, Cajal nevertheless overworked himself at the understaffed university, often teaching three classes per day, his schedule liable to last-minute changes. He spent his spare time at home, studying textbooks, mostly written in French, and practicing the histological techniques described by their authors, with scant equipment and without anyone to teach him. In this exhausted state, in the spring of 1878, a few months after the oposiciones disaster, Cajal went out one evening to a popular Zaragoza café, where he met a friend from his military days. Sitting outside in the garden, the two men were playing an intense game of chess, a favorite pastime of Cajal's that bordered on obsession. Absorbed in thought, contemplating his next move, he suddenly felt blood oozing up his throat, forcing him to cough, a condition that he diagnosed as a pulmonary hemorrhage. He finished the game, not wanting to alarm his friend or give way to panic.

Bloody coughing, symptomatic of a breach in the lungs, is a sign of tuberculosis. Also known as "phthsis" and "consumption," tuberculosis was a devastating scourge of the nineteenth century, killing from seventy to ninety percent of the urban population in Europe and North America by the late nineteenth century.[9] Although medical scientists rushed to save lives, many prominent figures in the Romantic movement glorified "the white death."[10] "It was the fashion to suffer from the lung," wrote Alexandre Dumas,[11] one of the favorite authors of Cajal's youth. Males between the ages of eighteen and thirty-five were known to be especially at risk, with the greatest exposure among soldiers stationed in close proximity to one another. Cajal was twenty-six years old, recently returned from Cuba, and bouts of malaria and dysentery had left his immune system vulnerable. He appeared to be a classic tubercular case. As a physician, he could ignore neither the diagnosis nor the prognosis: The death rate for patients with tuberculosis at the time was thought to be near one hundred percent.[12]

At the time, some doctors maintained that the only hope for recovery was through hydrotherapy, the use of water for healing. After two months of bed rest, Cajal set out for Panticosa, a spa town wedged against the base of the Pyrenees with a reputation for "marvelous baths."[13] Spanish physicians claimed that the natural presence of nitrogen in their waters helped to sedate the lungs.[14] An incurable Romantic, Cajal stubbornly rejected the advice of his doctors and sunk into a morbid despair, even contemplating suicide. However, while his fellow patients were dying, his condition started to improve, despite his desire to die. In time, he reversed course, deciding that he wanted to live.

Against every medical recommendation, he resumed a normal routine, exercising regularly and stimulating his mind with reading, art, and photography. He no longer carried himself as a tragic hero. Instead, trying to cleanse himself of poisonous negative thinking, he planted new thoughts in his mind, affirming his own survival. "Autocratically imposing itself over my lungs," Cajal writes in his autobiography, "my brains decreed that all was unjustified apprehension."[15] Cajal made an effort to refrain from fatalistic interpretation of his condition while his symptoms persisted. After a few months of willing himself to good health, he managed to recover and to return home. At that time, very few recovered from tuberculosis, and almost no one ever escaped the lethal clutches of the disease in a mere five months. The astonishing speed of Cajal's recovery has led even the most sympathetic biographers to suggest that his illness was, in fact, psychosomatic.[16]

Regardless of etiology, this experience of "disease" was Cajal's first direct encounter with psychology. Experimenting with himself as a subject, he learned firsthand the transformative power of what is called "auto-suggestion." Before even beginning his investigation of the structure of the brain, Cajal was exploring the dynamics of the mind. Although known for his purely anatomical research of the nervous system, "the father of modern neuroscience" initially was drawn to study the brain by an emotional attachment to his experience with psychology and the mind's potential to guide self-improvement. Cajal had been a patient in a sanitorium, in a state of acute distress. His dramatic, miraculous-seeming recovery, achieved through the power of conscious thought, inspired an alternative line of research[17] into morbid or anomalistic psychology, the study of seemingly paranormal effects based on rational and physical causes. At the end of his life, when Cajal left neurobiology and moved into hallucination, spiritism, and dreaming, he was returning to this persistent and personal mystical interest.

REFERENCES

1. Rallo et al., *Los sueños*, 51.
2. Cajal, *Recollections*, 211.
3. Irvin D. Yalom, *Existential Psychotherapy* (New York: Basic Books, 1980).
4. M. Khan and R. Masud, *Hidden Selves: Between Theory and Practice in Psychoanalysis* (London: Maresfield Library, 1988), 31.
5. Mark Solms, "An Introduction to the Neuroscientific Works of Sigmund Freud," in *The Pre-Psychoanalytic Writings of Sigmund Freud*, ed. Gertrudis Van de Vijver Gertrudis and Filip Geeradyn (London: Karnac Books, 2002), 17-35.
6. Laurence Simmons, *Freud's Italian Journey* (Amsterdam: Rodopi, 2006), 51.
7. Shepherd, *The Foundation of the Neuron Doctrine*, 66.
8. Cajal, *Recollections*, 252.
9. "Tuberculosis in Europe and North America, 1800–1922," in *Contagion: Historical Views of Diseases and Epidemics*, from the Harvard University Library Open Collections Program, http://ocp.hul.harvard.edu/contagion/tuberculosis.html.
10. John Frith, "History of Tuberculosis: Part 1—Phthsis, Consumption and the White Plague," *Journal of Military and Veterans' Health* 22, no. 2 (June 2014), 29–35.
11. René Jules Dubos and Jean Dubos, *The White Plague: Tuberculosis, Man, and Society* (New Brunswick, New Jersey: Rutgers University Press, 1952), 58.
12. "Tuberculosis in Europe and North America, 1800–1922"; Frith, "History of Tuberculosis: Part 1."
13. E. Littell, *Little's Living Age* (Boston: Little and Company, 1852), 373.
14. Albert Robin, "Treatment of Tuberculosis: Ordinary Therapeutics of Medical Men," trans. Léon Blanc (New York: Macmillan, 1913), 127.
15. Cajal, *Recollections*, 267.
16. Francisco Alonso Buron and Garcia Durán Muñoz. *Cajal: vida y obra*, 2nd edition (Barcelona: Editorial Científico-Médico, 1983), 103; Antonio Calvo Roy, *Cajal: Triunfar a toda costa* (Madrid: Alianza Editorial, 2007), 72.
17. Francisco López-Muñoz and Cecilio Álamo, "Los vínculos psiquiátricos en la obra y vida de Cajal," *Norte de Salud Mental* 8, no. 36 (2010), 71–83.

CHAPTER 6

✑

The Effects of Hypnosis
and Suggestion

Although Cajal was devoted to "the religion of the cell," there was an apocryphal strain of thought running through his research. For the last five years of his life, he abandoned his neurobiological research to focus almost exclusively on three manuscripts inspired by experimental psychology: *The Mysteries of the Tomb, The Hallucinations of Sleep,* and *Theories of Dreaming.*[1] Intrigued by parapsychology, the study of psychic phenomena, Cajal once invited a medium to live in his home in order to study her, before he realized that her effects were rooted in deception.[2] Cajal's dream project relates to his broader interest in what was called at the time *la psychologie nouvelle*—"the new psychology." In the second half of the nineteenth century, this influential movement cast occult phenomena such as human automatism, multiple personality, double consciousness, demonic possession, fugue states, faith cures, mediumship, and the effects of mental suggestion as topics for scientific investigation.[3] Cajal's intellectual development coincided with the gradual accommodation of mainstream discourse to include these radical themes. Even before studying neuroanatomy, Cajal conducted psychological experiments that shaped his understanding of the human mind. The history of parapsychology and its effect on nineteenth-century scientists informs Cajal's attitude toward dream work and illuminates the relationship between Cajal and Freud, who reacted differently to a similar intellectual climate.

It was another Viennese physician, Franz Anton Mesmer, who created the initial fervor that would spread throughout Europe. In the late eighteenth century, Mesmer adopted the technique of treating his patients

with magnets. According to Mesmer, the universe is an ocean of mag-
netic fluid, the disturbance of which caused disease. Through an invisible
force, which he called "animal magnetism," Mesmer claimed to generate
an artificial tide capable of restoring health to an individual. With his hair
clubbed back at the nape of his neck, in the fashion of a European gentle-
man, Mesmer sat in front of his patients, his knees touching theirs, as he
passed his hands over their limbs. Sometimes, Mesmer did not even need
to be present for this treatment. According to reports, Mesmer "was able
to influence people sitting in another room simply by pointing to their
images reflected in a mirror, even though these people could see him neither directly nor indirectly in the mirror."[4] His sensational cures became
public performances, attracting crowds that included Mozart and Marie
Antoinette. Mesmer always expected that it would be only a matter of
time before the scientific establishment recognized his discovery.

Animal magnetism seemed to tap into a darker reservoir of human
potential, at once astonishing and threatening. Mesmer was exiled to Paris,
where he managed to magnetize a roomful of two hundred people. When a
revolution broke out in Haiti, Mesmer credited animal magnetism, newly
introduced among the people, with unleashing their violent instincts. The
Marquis de Lafayette was a Mesmerist, and Mesmer hoped that he would
introduce animal magnetism to General George Washington. Whereas
the wife of King Louis XVI was a swooning believer, the king himself was
not, and in 1784 he appointed a commission to investigate the legitimacy
of animal magnetism. Then a diplomat in Paris, Benjamin Franklin issued
the commission's finding: Mesmerism did not qualify as a scientific theory because the effects "followed from an anticipated conviction, & could
have been an effect of the imagination."[5] No one could deny, however, that
this imaginary effect seemed to provide real benefits. "If the medicine of
imagination is the best," Mesmer's assistant argued, "why shouldn't we
practice it?"[6] This insight—that state of mind can influence the health
of the body—unites ancient healing practices with modern psychology,
with its theories of neurosis and hysteria, and even contemporary fields
of research, such as embodied cognition. Before there was a science of the
"unconscious," animal magnetism, or Mesmerism, exposed the hidden
power of the human mind to European civilization.

After the death of Mesmer, the next generation of Mesmerists moved
to separate animal magnetism from the mythological theories of their
founder. For example, the Marquis de Puységur, a French nobleman who
reportedly cured sixty-two out of three hundred peasants near his estate,
changed the name of the phenomenon to "artificial somnambulism"
because the altered state that his subjects were experiencing resembled
sleep. Puységur also magnetized objects, such as a rod or a tree, to imbue

them with healing powers. Interestingly, during the French Revolution, peasants would gather around those same trees, known as "liberty trees," to hear stirring political speeches.[7] This episode hints at the potential effects of animal magnetism as a means of social control. Puységur did not believe in magic trees, but he grasped the fundamentals of deeply-rooted belief. He explained,

> The entire doctrine of Animal magnetism is contained in the two words: *Believe* and *want*. I *believe* that I have the power to set into action the vital principle of my fellow-men; I *want* to make use of it; this is all my science and all my means.

The mind is prone to manipulation that can transform our experience of reality. "*Believe* and *want*, Sirs," said Puységur, "and you will do as much as I."[8] In the late nineteenth century, the future Nobel Laureate Charles Richet claimed that many of the developments in contemporary studies of mind in fact originated with the work of Puységur.[9]

Before reaching the scientific establishment, artificial somnambulism spread throughout the nineteenth century by traveling showmen, whose public demonstrations captivated audiences throughout Europe. In 1840, "public wonder worker" Charles Lafontaine visited London, where he proceeded to magnetize the lions at the city zoo. At the end of his tricks, like many a diligent magician, Lafontaine would invite skeptical audience members to the stage, especially doctors and scientists, to exorcise their doubts. One night James Braid, a Scottish surgeon still unconvinced by the phenomenon, attended Lafontaine's show in order to witness the scene for himself.[10] Braid saw that the effects of artificial somnambulism were real, but he did not believe in their causes. A scientific researcher in his own right, Braid designed experiments in which he would concentrate on an object at a certain height above his nose, at a certain distance from his face. With a concentrated gaze, he was able to produce the effects of artificial somnambulism. Magnetism was real, but there was no need for a magnetizer. Even without external agency, he demonstrated, the mind can transform itself.

Braid billed his version of magnetism as a new field: "neurohypnology," later shortened to "hypnotism." "Hypnotism," Braid said, "laid no claim to produce any phenomena which were not quite reconcilable with well-established physiological and psychological principles."[11] Hypnosis was acknowledged as a medical treatment after other surgeons demonstrated its effectiveness as an anesthetic. In the second half of the nineteenth century, the dream of Mesmer, though free of Mesmer and his theories, finally was realized: Rationalism and positivism dominated the intellectual discourse—"The rationale or doctrine of nervous sleep,"[12] in Braid's words, came to preoccupy many of the leading figures in medical science.

Cajal likely encountered this radical truth long before he became a doctor, not in a medical text but in a popular work of fiction. In Alexandre Dumas' 1844 novel,[13] the nineteen-year-old Edmund Dantes is imprisoned for a crime that he did not commit. In jail, he meets an elderly prisoner named Abbé Faria, whom Dumas modeled after a famous magnetist of the same name. Abbé Faria was a mysterious figure: Faria was born in the Portuguese province of Goa in India, claimed to be descended from Brahmins, took vows as a Catholic monk, and commanded a battalion of *sansculottes* during the French Revolution.[14] Like the fictional character in Dumas' novel, Faria was arrested and held in solitary confinement, which is where he allegedly discovered autosuggestion. In *The Count of Monte Cristo*, Dantes is on the verge of suicide before he befriends Faria, the so-called "mad priest" who becomes his teacher and reveals to the younger prisoner the location of a treasure on the island of Monte Cristo, which no one but Faria believes is real. Before he dies, Faria seems to acknowledge the influence of his suggestion in the mind of his impressionable comrade. As a teenager, feeling imprisoned by the tyrannical restrictions of his father, Cajal was captivated by *The Count of Monte Cristo*, which he stole from a neighbor's attic and read in secret, mesmerized by its pages.[15] He always was extraordinarily sensitive to fiction; books such as *Don Quixote* and *Robinson Crusoe* suggested to him archetypes and narratives that he would grow to imitate.

The suggestion of suggestibility—not consciously, of course—already was apparent to Cajal. After his will proved triumphant over the morbid atmosphere at Panticosa, he returned to Zaragoza a free man, driven by the force of this new aggressive program. While walking the streets of Zaragoza, Cajal saw a woman whose beauty instantly enchanted him, like an image of the Madonna in classical paintings. Her name was Silvería Fañanás. They became engaged to wed, but before he could marry her, he had to conduct another informal psychological experiment—"studying thoroughly the psychology of my fiancée, which turned out to be," he said, "the complement of my own."[16] With newfound confidence in his intellectual strengths, he published his first efforts at histological research. He refused a position at a rural hospital; his place, he maintained, was in the laboratory and not the clinic. Raised in poverty and accustomed to sacrifice, he was prepared for the reduced financial prospects that were the inevitable consequences of his decision. He spent whatever extra resources were available on laboratory equipment, including foreign textbooks and journals. His new wife had no problem sacrificing to adapt to this course; she assumed complete responsibility for the household and, in the final tally, their seven children. Cajal was determined to make himself into a biological researcher, to challenge the foreign masters, and to glorify himself and his country. The idea was seeded in his mind, that he was an heroic scientific investigator, a belief that he would reaffirm continuously through his professional career with the determination of a certain vengeful prisoner.

Freud already was an established biological researcher, with similarly grand scientific ambitions. After considerable success, he had reason to believe that neuroanatomy would yield the breakthrough discovery that he ardently desired. After earning his doctorate from the University of Vienna in 1881, Freud continued his research in Brücke's physiological institute, where he had worked off and on for years. For Freud, as for Cajal, romantic love would profoundly affect the course of his professional life. Freud was twenty-six years old when he fell in love with Martha Bernays. He desperately wanted to marry her, but he did not have the requisite financial or social capital to satisfy her prominent family. Brücke, who was like a father to Freud, offered him some surprising advice: Leave the laboratory. There was no money in anatomical research, Brücke said. Moreover, there were two other assistants in the laboratory who, equally talented and promising but older and, moreover, not Jewish, stood in the way of his promotion. In 1882, after years of fruitful research under a beloved mentor, Freud made the difficult and fateful decision to leave the Physiological Institute at University of Vienna, his alma mater, to become a junior resident at the Vienna General Hospital. Shuffling between surgery, internal medicine, and psychiatry, he was unsure of the field in which he wanted to specialize until eventually he settled into neurology and psychiatry.[17]

Freud's departure from the physiology laboratory happened to coincide with acceptance of hypnosis into the scientific establishment, when Jean-Martin Charcot presented his theory of *grand hypnotism* before the National Academy of Sciences. In his famed clinic at Salpêtrière, Charcot, "the Napoleon of neuroses," studied thousands of patients diagnosed with neurological diseases and came to the conclusion that hypnotizability in a patient was a sign of underlying neuropathology.[18] These ideas formed the basis of the Salpêtrière school of hypnotism, whereas a competing school, championed by Ambroise-Auguste Liébault and Hippolyte Bernheim, sprang from a clinic in Nancy and maintained that susceptibility to hypnosis was not a form of pathology but, rather, a general effect of suggestion. Cajal sided with the Nancy doctrine of universal suggestibility,[19] whereas Freud was persuaded by Charcot's demonstration that hypnosis was both a sign of and a treatment for mental illness. Thus, the two explorers of the mind reacted differently to their shared intellectual environment, and their ideological separation widened into divergent approaches that persist today.

Freud continued to publish articles on neuroanatomy in the *Proceedings of the Imperial Academy of Sciences* and elsewhere. In his 1884 review, "The Structure of the Elements of the Nervous System," he discusses nerve fibrils—the thin, delicate strands that run in every direction throughout the length of nerves. Freud neither addresses the continuity of nerves nor challenges the reticular theory; rather, he confirms the internal composition of the nerve cell, which is a different matter. In a technical paper from the same year, Freud introduces a new histological stain, "gold chloride," which allowed him to see the inner workings of living cells,[20] revealing unprecedented subtlety of detail. With this technique, Freud intended to trace the fibers of the brain in both adults and embryos in the hope of answering the greatest question at the vanguard of neuroanatomy: What is the relationship *between* the nerves? Had he committed himself to finding the answer, he might well have secured his fame in neuroscience.[21]

Curiously, while Freud's work brought him to the edge of neuroscience, Cajal's interests took him to the heart of hypnosis. Books and articles on hypnosis started to appear in Spanish translation in the 1880s,[22] and Cajal also was able to read French. Initially, he started probing this field through a series of science fiction short stories, later published under the pseudonym Dr. Bacteria. One of these tales, "The Fabricator of Honor," is about a hypnotist, Dr. Alejandro Mirahonda (whose surname means "look" and "deep" in Spanish),[23] who was educated in Germany and France and is the darling of Bernheim and the Nancy school. "With very little effort," the narrator says, Mirahonda "could create negative and positive hallucinations, metamorphoses and dissociations of the personality, and all sorts of sensory and motor phenomena, not just in hysterics, but even in sane, alert individuals."[24] Mirahonda tells the inhabitants of a rural town that he possesses a morality vaccine that will change their behavior, accentuating virtue and eliminating vice. Cajal's allegory amplifies the effects of suggestion, thereby suggesting that human beings are prone to social, religious, or political suggestion from an authoritarian figure. These stories represent experiments of his imagination in which Cajal starts to work through some of his ideas about the power of suggestion. The narrator of the story—possibly Cajal himself—concludes that suggestion is necessary to maintain order and to restrain our animal instincts in order to progress.

While Cajal was conducting fictional experiments, Freud was observing the use of hypnosis on actual patients. Freud had heard of Charcot's work on neuroses when, in 1885, he received a grant to study the Salpêtrière. Although the anatomy of the nervous system was still his stated concern—the official subject of his research was to be pathological lesions in infantile brains—Freud was drawn to the commanding presence of Charcot and to his compelling ideas. In a letter to Martha, Freud refers to Charcot as "one of the greatest of physicians and a man whose common sense borders on genius."[25] After approximately a month, Freud complained to Martha that he wanted to return home early, in part because he did not have enough contact with Charcot. In time, however, Freud was able to form a personal relationship with Charcot, who would influence his life profoundly. High on cocaine, after one of Charcot's celebrated parties,[26] Freud giddily recalls that Charcot kissed him on the forehead. "No other human being has ever affected me in the same way," Freud writes.[27] He later named his first son "Jean-Martin," after his idol.[28]

Through his legendary demonstrations of hypnotic technique, Charcot opened Freud's eyes to the science of the future, and so Freud would leave neuroanatomy behind because it seemed to him to be the science of the past. When he returned to Vienna, Freud established a psychiatric practice, announcing his consulting hours in the newspaper. He could not yet afford the travel fare for house calls, but he needed the revenue from private patients. More established specialists in Vienna would send Freud a steady stream of wealthy neurotics, and Freud would employ the controversial new French techniques, including hypnosis, which he learned at the Salpêtrière.[29] After his study abroad, he translated Charcot's "Tuesday Lectures," which deal with hypnosis and the etiology of hysteria, into German. During Freud's entire career as a psychoanalyst, a portrait of Charcot and the Salpêtrière clinic hung above his iconic couch.[30] When the neuroanatomist Theodor Meynert, his former director at the hospital, suggested that he return to the hospital to take control of the department, Freud declined.[31]

Interestingly, at the same time that Freud was starting to incorporate hypnosis into his practice, Cajal started to experiment with hypnosis for himself. While serving as the Chair of Anatomy at the University of Valencia, Cajal organized what he sardonically named the "Committee for Psychological Investigation" with some of his friends and colleagues.[32] Converting the small apartment that he shared with his wife and five children into a clinic, he used hypnosis to treat "the most remarkable kinds of hysterics, neuraesthenics, maniacs, and even accredited spiritualistic mediums." With these techniques, he was able to produce total or partial amnesia, to expose the presence of multiple personalities, and to evoke remembrances of the forgotten past. Cajal claims to have cured depression, to have returned phobic eaters to their regular diets, to have enabled those with hysterical paralysis to walk again, and to have aided the erasure of painful memories. Most important, he confirmed the Nancy school hypothesis by hypnotizing normal and healthy individuals as well. Cajal's only scientific publication on hypnosis concerned its analgesic effects on a woman who was terrified of the pains associated with her sixth childbirth. The makeshift nature of Cajal's research is highlighted by the fact that this "robust, tranquil, rather lymphatic–hyperaemic woman"[33] was his wife, Silvería. Cajal briefly considered clinical practice, drawn as Freud had been toward the new frontier, but Cajal did not believe that his research in hypnosis was original, and ultimately he was ambivalent about its moral consequences.

Reflecting on the effects of hypnosis, Cajal felt a mixture of surprise and disillusionment—"surprise at recognizing the reality of phenomena of cerebral automatism deemed thitherto tricks and deceptions of circus magicians" and "sad disillusionment that the human brain, which is so highly lauded, the 'masterpiece of creation,' suffers from the enormous defect of suggestibility."[34] "The masterpiece of creation" was a common epithet for the brain; to Cajal, the human brain represented the apex of logic and reasoning, refined throughout eons of evolution. Suggestion threatened to undermine our higher mental function and sabotage our conscious will, which Cajal exalted. "If there is anything truly divine in us," he would say later, "it is the will."[35] This will, which he believed to be responsible for his "miraculous" recovery from illness, was threatened by the subversive power of suggestion. Throughout his career, he would rely on his will to sustain decades of arduous and largely independent research and to drive him through failure and hardships on the way to his breakthrough discoveries. Cajal even went as far as to assert that the reticular theorists, especially his rival Camillo Golgi, were clinging to their defunct model of the nervous system because of erroneous suggestion. From Cajal's point of view, the power of suggestion to mislead great minds spelled peril for scientific thinking and constituted a major threat to his entire ethos. Therefore, when he called Freud's theories the product of suggestion, Cajal was not only dismissing their scientific value but also passing a moral and intellectual judgment on the man who invented them.

It is worth mentioning that parapsychology—or "psychical research"—was not the only intriguing new opportunity that Cajal spurned. In 1885, a cholera epidemic in Valencia claimed more than one hundred and twenty thousand lives.[36] Although many of his neighbors were stricken with the disease, Cajal and his family remained unharmed. Generally, the younger generation believed that the disease was caused by bacteria, only recently discovered, whereas older physicians thought that the cause was bad air. The provincial government asked Cajal to investigate the origin of the disease. In a monograph, he confirms the bacterial hypothesis, and he recommended a vaccine, which he tested successfully. Importantly, he refused financial reward, fearing that money would taint his research; his only compensation was a new microscope gratefully donated by the authorities. Like Freud at the physiological institute, Cajal was faced with a career decision: He could have diverted his course toward the promising and potentially more lucrative field of bacteriology, in which he had found some success. However, whereas he saw the bacterium as the persistent villain of our evolutionary narrative, he saw the cell as its enduring hero. For the rest of his life—with the notable exception of his final psychological works, including the book on dreams—Cajal would, humbling and unsparingly, devote himself to the religion of the cell.

After his experiments with hypnosis and suggestion, Cajal experienced a microscopic revelation. In 1887, he visited the Madrid laboratory of Luis Simarro, a neuropsychiatrist who had recently returned from the Salpêtrière, where he had studied psychiatry under Charcot, as well as anatomy and histology with the experts in those fields. Simarro would have told Cajal about all of his experiences abroad, but the stories of hypnosis no longer interested him; he only cared to learn about any new histological techniques, one of which was *the black reaction*. In fact, the black reaction was not new at all; almost fifteen years earlier, the Italian anatomist Camillo Golgi had invented the stain in a supply closet of the local mental hospital that he directed. For some reason, which is still unknown, the "Golgi stain," a preparation based on the compound silver nitrate, exposes a small percentage of nervous elements, highlighting some fibers while leaving others uncolored. However, the scientific community had all but abandoned the stain, which proved erratic and appeared not to provide any groundbreaking information. The textbooks that Cajal read hardly mentioned the black reaction, but he was awestruck by Simarro's demonstration of its use and was fascinated by the stark, ink-colored spindles on a translucent yellow background. More than that, he suddenly realized that the material of the mind might be illuminated once and for all. "Here everything is simple," Cajal remembers, "clear without confusion. Nothing more to interpret."[37] He resolved to apply the stain to the brain in order to clarify the fundamental questions in neuroanatomy. "To know the brain," he claimed idealistically, "is equivalent to ascertaining the material course of thought and will." The object of psychology finally was at hand; "The dream technique is a reality!"[38]

Inspired, Cajal returned to Valencia and started his investigations of the nervous system. He managed to improve the black reaction in crucial ways that allowed him to provide convincing evidence for independent nerve cells, whose existence he repeatedly demonstrated in different regions of the brain in different animals. Cajal rushed to publish these results, sending copies of his papers to all the leading experts. No one responded; there were no foreign scientists who spoke Spanish. Therefore, Cajal decided to present his findings in person at the International Congress of Anatomy in Berlin, traveling at his own expense with his microscopes and slides in his suitcase. A nobody, at the time, outside of Spain, he nervously corralled the greatest neuroanatomists in the world and, in halting French, struggled to get them see the true structure of an individual nerve cell for the first time. Eventually, he won them over. The new facts were clear and startling enough that the elder statesman, Albert von Kölliker, promised immediately to learn Spanish strictly in order read Cajal's work. This is the moment when Santiago Ramón y Cajal, the unknown researcher from provincial Spain, fatefully became known as "Cajal."[39] The field of neuroanatomy would never be the same. Notably, there was one neuroanatomist absent from the historic proceedings: Sigmund Freud.

Two months before the Berlin anatomy conference, Freud attended the First International Congress of Psychology, held in Paris. The event was organized by Theodule Ribot, the French psychologist and leader of *la psychologie nouvelle.* Jean-Martin Charcot was the official president of the congress, which featured important participants from around the world, including Hippolyte Bernheim, Charles Richet, Wilhelm Wundt, Pierre Janet, and William James. The entire second session was devoted to the subject of hypnotism.[40] The amateur hypnotist Cajal might have been there, as well, had he not chosen histology over hysteria. Despite their shared interests, Cajal was at home with the neuroanatomists, and Freud had joined ranks with the experimental psychologists.

The career paths of Santiago Ramón y Cajal and Sigmund Freud now had diverged permanently. Despite his interest in experimental psychology and his personal experience with hypnosis and suggestion, Cajal experienced a conversion to neurohistology that resembled an awakening. His visual sense, the preeminent way in which he engaged with the world around him, was stimulated by the picture of stained brain tissue beneath a microscope. More than anything else, he saw in the anatomy of the nervous system the potential answer to a timeless question: What is the source of mental life? While parapsychology intrigued him and bacteriology tempted him, his dedication to anatomy was deeper and more abiding. On the other hand, although Freud was a promising and successful neuroanatomist, with lofty ambitions in that discipline, the more practical considerations of his personal life led him away from the laboratory.

REFERENCES

1. Cannon, *Explorer*, 261; Rallo et al., *Los sueños*, 14.
2. Cannon, *Explorer*, 261.
3. Makari, *Revolution*, 48.

4. Henri F. Ellenberger, *The Discovery of the Unconscious: The History and Evolution of Dynamic Psychiatry* (New York: Basic Books, 1970).

5. Douglas J. Lanska and Joseph T. Lanska, "Franz Anton Mesmer and the Rise of Animal Magnetism," in *Brain, Mind and Medicine: Neuroscience in the 18th Century*, ed. Harry Whitaker, C. U. M. Smith, and Stanley Finger (New York: Springer, 2007), 310.

6. Lanska and Lanska, "Franz Anton Mesmer and the Rise of Animal Magnetism," 316.

7. Ellenberger, *Discovery of the Unconscious*, 73.

8. Ellenberger, *Discovery of the Unconscious*, 72.

9. Ellenberger, *Discovery of the Unconscious*, 74.

10. Ellenberger, *Discovery of the Unconscious*, 82.

11. Judith Pintar and Steven J. Lynn, *Hypnosis: A Brief History* (Hoboken, New Jersey: Wiley-Blackwell, 2008), 45.

12. Pintar and Lynn, *Hypnosis: A Brief History*, 45.

13. Alexandre Dumas, *The Count of Monte Cristo*, trans. Peter Washington (New York: Knopf, 2009).

14. Lee Siegel, *Trance-Migrations: Stories of India, Tales of Hypnosis* (Chicago: University of Chicago Press, 2014), 85.

15. Cajal, *Recollections*, 101.

16. Cajal, *Recollections*, 270.

17. "The Young Physician," in *The Freud Encyclopedia: Theory, Therapy, and Culture*, ed. Edward Erwin (New York: Routledge, 2002), 221.

18. "People and Discoveries: Jean-Martin Charcot 1825–1893," *A Science Odyssey*, PBS. org, http://www.pbs.org/wgbh/aso/databank/entries/bhchar.html.

19. Cajal, *Recollections*, 313; López-Muñoz et al., "The Neurobiological Interpretation of the Mental Functions in the Work of Santiago Ramón y Cajal," 8.

20. Solms, "Introduction to the Neuroscientific Works of Sigmund Freud," 20; Simo Køppe, "The Psychology of the Neuron: Freud, Cajal and Golgi," *Scandinavian Journal of Psychology* 24 (1983), 8; Lazaros Triarhou and Manuel D. Cerro, "Freud's Contribution to Neuroanatomy," *Archives of Neurology* 42 (March 1985), 285.

21. See Frank Sulloway, *Freud, Biologist of the Mind: Beyond the Psychoanalytic Legend* (New York: Basic Books, 1970); Lazaros C. Triarhou, "Exploring the Mind with a Microscope: Freud's Beginnings in Neurobiology," *Hellenic Journal of Psychology* 6 (2009), 1–13.

22. José Sala, Etzel Cardeña, María Carmen Holgado, et al., "The Contributions of Ramón y Cajal and Other Spanish Authors to Hypnosis," *Internation Journal of Clinical and Experimental Hypnosis* 56, no. 4 (2008), 361–372; see p. 362.

23. Laura Otis, *Membranes: Metaphors of Invasion in Nineteenth-Century Literature, Science, and Politics* (Baltimore: Johns Hopkins University Press, 1999): 75.

24. Cajal, *Vacation Stories*, 40.

25. Sigmund Freud, "Letter 86," in *Letters of Sigmund Freud*, ed. Ernst L. Freud, trans. Tania Stern and James Stern (New York: Dover, 1992), 185.

26. Howard Markel, *An Anatomy of Addiction: Sigmund Freud, William Halstead, and the Miracle Drug, Cocaine* (New York: Vintage Books, 2012), 125.

27. Markel, *An Anatomy of Addiction*, 125.

28. "Jean-Martin Charcot: 1825–1893," *A Science Odyssey: People and Discoveries*, PBS. org, http://www.pbs.org/wgbh/aso/databank/entries/bhchar.html.

29. Solms, "Introduction to the Neuroscientific Works of Sigmund Freud."

30. "4378" in Collections, *Freud Museum London* https://www.freud.org.uk/about/collections/detail/76154.

31. Hubert Van Hoorde, "Freud's Merit as a Psychiatrist," in *The Pre-Psychoanalytic Writings of Sigmund Freud*, ed. Gertrudis Van de Vijver Gertrudis and Filip Geeradyn (London: Karnac Books, 2002), 49.

32. Cajal, *Recollections*, 312.

33. Lazaros C. Triarhou et al., "Cajal's Brief Experimentation with Suggestion," *Journal of the History of the Neurosciences* 16, no. 4 (October 2007), 355.

34. Cajal, *Recollections*, 315.

35. Benjamin Ehrlich, "Santiago Ramón y Cajal: Café Chats," *New England Review* 33, no. 1 (2012), 182.

36. "The Cholera in Spain," *The New York Times* (June 20, 1890), 4.

37. Marco Piccolino, Enrica Strettoi, and Elena Laurenzi, "Santiago Ramón y Cajal, the Retina and the Neuron Theory," *Documenta Opthalmologica* 71, no. 2 (1989), 123–141; p. 123.

38. Piccolino, Strettoi, and Laurenzi, "Santiago Ramón y Cajal, the Retina and the Neuron Theory," 123.

39. Cajal, *Recollections*, 357.

40. International Congress of Physiological Psychology, August 6–10, 1889, Paris, France, adapted from M. Rosenzweig, W. Holtzman, M., Sabourin, and D. Bélanger, *History of the International Union of Psychological Science* (Hove, UK: Psychology Press, 2000), .

CHAPTER 7

◦◦◦

On the Divergence of Psychology
and Neuroanatomy

Freud's career in neurohistology effectively ended in 1888, the "year of fortune" in which Cajal's career auspiciously began.[1] Freud ceased to explore questions of brain anatomy for their own sake, unless such research might produce pathological or psychological insights. However, on the subject of his relationship to Cajal, we might ask, How did Freud respond to Cajal's new discoveries? The only writings of Freud's that deal explicitly with the structure of the nerve cell come in the form of encyclopedia articles, written for hire and published anonymously. These records, which are not included in his collected works and have been exhumed only recently, reflect Freud's knowledge of the state of neuroanatomy at that time. Many biographers contend that Freud either preempted or at least presaged the tenets of the neuron theory.[2] However, the evidence suggests that he was in fact neither a pioneer of the theory nor among its earlier adopters.

In an article titled "Das Gehirn" ("The Brain"), one of his two contributions to a contemporary dictionary of medicine, Freud unequivocally confirms the reticular theory, stating that "the functioning elements of the nervous system form a complete unbroken net."[3] Because no one in the neuroanatomy community was aware of Cajal's groundbreaking work before 1889, at the earliest, it would not be fair to criticize Freud for this view. However, history shows that certain investigators did preempt or influence Cajal, finding evidence against the reticular theory and even suggesting the independence of the nerve cell. Freud is not among them. For example, just in the year prior to Cajal's findings, Wilhelm His, Auguste Forel, and Fritdjof Nansen each had challenged the reticular theory with ingenious methods: His examined hundreds of embryonic brains and suggested that their nerve fibers lacked continuity; Forel lesioned certain fibers and observed that the damage did not spread throughout the system, which implied the absence of continuity; and in his doctoral dissertation, Nansen reported the absence of anastomoses in the nervous system of marine animals.[4] Although his substantial contributions to neuroscience often are unheralded,[5] Freud did not participate in the ground-level construction of the neuron theory. This did not result from ineptitude but, rather, a lack of interest.

Even if Freud himself did not end up producing new evidence about nerve cell connections, he had ample opportunity to incorporate new facts on the subject that others, most notably Cajal, had revealed. Cajal's work, written in French, was published in German journals.[6] His neuroanatomy investigations were guided in part by a textbook written by Theodor Meynert, Freud's mentor at the Institute for Brain Anatomy. Freud likely was exposed to the same information as Cajal, with perhaps even better tools to explore the field. However, his attention had shifted elsewhere. The majority of his publications during this period dealt with hypnotism and suggestion, the methods that he learned at Salpêtrière. Their different foci at this time widen the gap between them further, creating a gulf between neurobiology and psychoanalysis that can still be perceived today.

Although the new discoveries in neuroanatomy might have flown under Freud's radar for a few years, the changes in the landscape became unmistakable when, in 1891, the anatomist Wilhelm Waldeyer published an influential review summarizing the new findings in neuroanatomy, mainly by Cajal, and proposing a coherent neuron doctrine, establishing the independent nerve cell as the anatomical, physiological, anabolic, metabolic, and genetic unit of the nervous system.[7] By 1892, hundreds of scientists had replaced the reticular theory with the neuron theory and were integrating this new vision of the structure and function of the brain into their work.[8] Although not an explicit denier, like Camillo Golgi, Freud does not appear to have assimilated the new views about the structure of the nervous system into his thinking.

It was not until 1893, in an article on organic paralysis, that Freud mentions the new theory and cites Cajal by name. "The modern histology of the nervous system," Freud writes, "[is] founded on the work of Golgi, Ramon y Cajal, Kölliker, etc."[9] This syntax raises doubts about Freud's knowledge of contemporary neuroanatomy: No active brain scientist would join the rivals Cajal and Golgi on the same side of this crucial scientific debate. For reasons unknown, though Freud spent five years preparing the article, this fact was not corrected.[10] It was not until another unsigned entry in an atlas of the brain—six years after Cajal demonstrated the anatomical independence of the nerve cell, five years after his findings were diffused within the German-speaking scientific community, and three years after the formal establishment of the neuron theory—that Freud finally acknowledged the existence of the neuron by referencing "the opposing views of Golgi and Ramon [y Cajal] on the structure of the nervous tissue."[11]

To Freud, knowledge of neuroanatomy was useful only to the extent that it might aid him in addressing human psychology and psychopathology. In 1895, he started to work on a grandiose synthesis of our understanding of the mind and brain that he calls "Psychology for Neurologists." "I have never before experienced such a high degree of preoccupation," Freud says in a letter, part of a series exchanged with his friend and colleague Wilhelm Fleiss. "For two weeks I have been in the throes of a writing fever, believing that I had found the secret," he writes in another.[12] Presenting psychology as a natural science, Freud attempts to integrate all of his scientific experiences, from neuroanatomy and neurohistology, through clinical neurology and psychiatry, to parapsychology and experimental psychology. He wishes to combine his "quantity (Qn) theory," conceived through observations of neurotics and hysterics, with the "new knowledge of neuron[s]," which finally he has come to grasp. "The essence of this new knowledge," Freud writes, "is that the neuronic system consists of distinct but similarly constructed neuron[s] which only have contact with one another through an intervening foreign substance."[13] He saw in this revelation the anatomical and physiological evidence to support a scientific theory of the psyche.

Cocaine use perhaps contributed to the intensity of his mood swings over the next few months,[14] as he felt "alternately proud and overjoyed and ashamed and miserable" about his work. At one point he dropped "the whole business," only to pick it up once again. "Everything seemed to fall into place, the cogs meshed," he writes later, "and I had the impression that the thing now really was a machine that shortly would function on its own." Only soon thereafter, he refuses to share the work with Fleiss because to do so would be "like sending a six-month foetus to a ball."[15] Finally defeated, he throws the manuscript in a drawer and refuses to talk further about it, "no longer able to understand the state of mind in which [he] hatched the psychology."[16] After his death, that manuscript was recovered and published as *The Project for Scientific Psychology*.[17] Freud began his efforts with neurohistology, became fascinated by hypnosis and pathologies of the mind, moved into the realm of scientific psychology, and finally attempted to incorporate all of his prior research, including the anatomy of the brain, into one grand unified theory. With the failure of this project, he definitively abandoned the cell as a means to explain the psyche.

By the turn of the twentieth century, both the professional fates of Cajal and Freud were sealed. In 1899, Cajal was invited by the American psychologist G. Stanley Hall to participate in the decennial celebration of Clark University, where he showed histological drawings of the cerebral cortex.[18] That year, he published the first volume of his seminal *The Texture of the Nervous System*, in which he describes the structure of the nervous system and its evolution in different species. Among the references, he cites Freud and his 1884 work with the gold chloride method.[19] However, the Freud whom he cited no longer existed as a neuroanatomist. Ten years later, G. Stanley Hall invited Freud to the centennial celebration of Clark University, where he delivered "Five Lectures on Psychoanalysis," a landmark moment in the dissemination of Freudian theory and the basis for Ortega's popularizing 1911 article.[20] This was the closest that the two men came to sharing a stage.

The relationship between Cajal and Freud, defined by both intellectual familiarity and distance, seems to reflect the subsequent disconnect between neurobiology and psychoanalysis.[21] Although there have been collaborative and conciliatory efforts between the two disciplines, considerable philosophical and methodological differences remain. One of the current battlefronts for their ideological conflict happens to be the science of dreams.[22] For decades, two prominent researchers, J. Allan Hobson and Mark Solms, have been arguing with each other about the physiology of dreaming. More than anyone else, Hobson carries forward the mission of Cajal as a dream researcher, a neurobiologist who is intent upon disqualifying Freud and his theories.[23] In contrast, Solms is a psychoanalyst, at work on new translations of Freud, who claims to prove a number of Freud's theories through neurobiological research. Hobson argues that dreams are ad hoc frameworks for meaningless signals, whereas Solms uses physiological evidence to argue that dreams are indeed the expressions of wish-fulfillment. Each interprets certain patterns of brain activity and associates the changes with dreaming. Their fascinating debate, and the illuminating world of contemporary dream research, is beyond the scope of this work. Symbolically, however, their findings are crucial to this discussion. Hobson and Solms, proxies for Cajal and Freud, have each proposed an origin of dreaming in the brain: Both are located in the ventral–tegmental area of the brain, separated by a few centimeters,[24] just this close and that far.

REFERENCES

1. Cajal, *Recollections*, 321.
2. Køppe, "The Psychology of the Neuron, 9.

3. Køppe, "The Psychology of the Neuron," 8.
4. Bentivoglio and Mazzarello, "The Anatomical Foundations of Clinical Neurology," 162.
5. Solms, "Introduction to the Neuroscientific Works of Sigmund Freud," 17.
6. Merchán et al., *Cajal and De Castro's Neurohistological Methods*, 6.
7. Shepherd, *The Foundation of the Neuron Doctrine*, 182.
8. Køppe, "The Psychology of the Neuron," 9.
9. Køppe, "The Psychology of the Neuron," 9.
10. Køppe, "The Psychology of the Neuron," 9.
11. Lazaros Triarhou, "A Review of Edward Flatau's 1894 Atlas of the Human Brain by the Neurologist Sigmund Freud," *European Neurology* 65 (2011), 10–15, https://www.karger.com/Article/FullText/322500.
12. J. M. Masson, ed., *The Complete Letters of Sigmund Freud to Wilhelm Fliess, 1887–1904* (Cambridge, Massachusetts: Harvard University Press, 1985), excerpts.
13. Freud, *Project for a Scientific Psychology*, 358, http://users.clas.ufl.edu/burt/freud%20fleiss%20letters/200711781-013.pdf.
14. Chapter 1 in David Cohen, *Freud on Coke* (London: Cutting Edge Press, 2012).
15. Rivka Warshawsky, "The Symptom as Metaphor: Freud's 'Project'," in *The Pre-Psychoanalytic Writings of Freud*, 171–172.
16. Warshawsky, "The Symptom as Metaphor," 171–172.
17. Volume 1 in *The Complete Psychological Works*.
18. Duane E. Haines, "Santiago Ramón y Cajal at Clark University, 1899: His Only Visit to the United States," *Brain Research Reviews* 55, no. 2 (October 1, 2007), 463–480.
19. Cajal, *Histology*, 24.
20. Rallo et al., *Los sueños*, 20–21.
21. See Chapter 1, note 6.
22. Køppe, "The Psychology of the Neuron," 9.
23. See Rachel Aviv, Rachel. "Hobson's Choice: Can Freud's Theory of Dreams Hold Up Against Modern Neuroscience?" *The Believer* (October 2007); J. Allan Hobson, *Dreaming and the Brain* (New York: Basic Books, 1989), 36; G. William Domhoff, "Refocusing the Neurocognitive Approach to Dreams; A Critique of the Hobson Versus Solms Debate," *Dreaming* 15 (2005), 3–20.
24. Domhoff, "Refocusing the Neurocognitive Approach to Dreams," 3–20.

CHAPTER 8

ⱱⱱ

Cajal's Psyche and His Readings of Freud

Although both Freud and Cajal received similar training and entertained similar scientific ambitions, Freud grew to be Cajal's foil. Cajal saw Freud as a defector from neuroanatomy; he could not understand why Freud chose psychology over biology, because he himself had not. In Cajal's religion of the cell, Freud was a raving heretic, a theoretical upstart who impatiently undermined the primacy of empirical fact. To Cajal's careful cultivation of Spanish neurobiology, Freud was an invasive species, threatening to infect young scientific minds through rampant suggestion, preying on the atavism of the imperfect human brain. Freud's talent and promise, to Cajal's disappointment, were wasted in pursuit of pseudoscientific theory, and the stubborn popularity of his theories left Cajal irritated and perplexed.

Yet, to quote Ortega's assessment of Freud, "rather than false," this interpretation of Cajal's reaction to Freud "[is] not true."[1] If the need to intervene against Freud's intellectual contagion were that urgent, Cajal would have published more in refutation, including the evidence from his diary. We are faced with the contradiction that although he was openly disdainful of Freud and talked for years about disproving him, Cajal decided to remain publicly silent. He neither confronted Freud nor directly dismissed him. Instead, for sixteen years, without interruption, Cajal carried on, in this private diary, a shadow conversation that lasted right until the point of his death. Therefore, the question is, Why did Cajal spend so much of his time intimately engaged with someone he claims to have hated?[2]

In the late stages of his life, Cajal was mired in a fierce pessimism.[3] Throughout his career, the potential for self-improvement made possible by neuronal plasticity was a source of motivational energy for Cajal. However, his research into the degeneration and regeneration of the nervous system challenged Cajal with a deeply resonant question: Young cells certainly regenerate, but do older cells as well? The prospect of regeneration was vital to Cajal's spirit. He was awed by the persistence and creativity displayed in the developing neuron's response to trauma. Cajal carried this idea of plasticity further, defining intellectual character as the ceaseless ability to change one's opinions. Moreover, Cajal, as an leading representative of the Generation of '98, dedicated himself to the regeneration of Spanish culture in the aftermath of the collective trauma of the Spanish–American war.[4] In one of the only instances of misinterpretation about the neuron,[5] Cajal, on the cusp of old age, saw the harsh reality of his own mortality in the fixity of older neurons. "Once the development has ended," Cajal concludes, "the founts of growth and regeneration of the dendrites dried up irrevocably. In the adult centers, the nerve paths are something fixed, ended, and immutable. Everything may die, nothing may be regenerated."[6]

This was Cajal's state of mind when, at sixty-six years of age, he started to record his dream diary. As his health declined, he began a slow and pained withdrawal from the surrounding world.[7] One afternoon, after his customary *tertulia*, he complained of a debilitating headache, which worsened with any exposure to noise. A few minutes of sustained attention caused what he described as unbearable pressure in his brain, once the sovereign organ of thought and will, capable of twenty consecutive hours of "cerebral polarity," a state of total and relentless concentration on an object of study.[8] Cajal's friend and former studentt Dr. Nicolás Achúcarro diagnosed him with cerebral arteriosclerosis, a constriction of blood vessels in the brain that leads to a lack of oxygen. Some have suggested that, like his earlier bout with tuberculosis, this may have been a psychosomatic ailment. Again, regardless of etiology of his condition, it is important to note that in his mind, Cajal was suffering from disease associated with senility, which affected not his body but, rather, his brain. Others wondered if the neurons of the great neuroscientist were deteriorating.[9]

The doctors recommended that he remain in silence, without speaking or listening to conversation. This inaugurated a difficult period for Cajal, who was used to a tightly controlled routine and a robust schedule of activities. He stopped attending tertulias, vital to his daily functioning for forty years. Whereas natural beauty always had a healing effect on him, the doctors now advised him to either stay indoors or carry a parasol, which may have blocked the sun's rays but exposed him to the pitying glances of passersby. As time went on, any walk of more than a few hundred meters exhausted him, and he was forced to ride in a car, which he hated. Eventually, Cajal retreated to his cellar, where he installed a small laboratory, a writing desk, and a library of thousands of books.[10] Visiting friends and colleagues nicknamed this place "The Cave."[11] While his days were less enjoyable without his favorite activities, his nights were insufferable. Chronic insomnia troubled him to such an extent that he resorted to sedatives as potent as morphine. Those who knew Cajal at this time in his life testified that he became obsessed with thoughts of death.

Although framed as an intellectual project aimed at disproving a theory, Cajal's dream diary was deeply personal, as its writing spans a period during which he was acutely depressed.[12] Distressing events loom in the background of his entries. For example, in 1922, at seventy years of age, Cajal was required by law to retire from his university professorship. Outwardly, he did not seem upset, accepting the change in stride. However, having occupied faculty positions and taught students for forty years, he experienced a radical and sudden loss to his social and professional identity. Without telling anyone, he chose not to attend his final class at the university for fear of being overwhelmed publically by emotion—the "madwoman of the house"[13]—which would have been intolerable. Cajal shied away from the many honors and tributes that poured in. When he was named an honorary rector of the university, Cajal declined to attend the ceremony. When the King of Spain organized a celebration of Cajal, as the French nation had celebrated Pasteur, Cajal failed to attend. The Spanish Senate planned a tribute but, once again, he absented himself. We can imagine the psychological burden of all these avoidances. "Man can, if he is so determined, become the sculptor of his own brain,"[14] the famous Cajal quote goes. After 1926, when the government unveiled an ornate toga-clad sculpture of Cajal by the park path he most loved to walk, he never walked there again. He wanted to be the sculptor, not the lifeless stone.

Toward the end of Cajal's life, a poignant episode caught him by surprise and revealed the emotional undercurrent of his behavior. Once, while working in The Cave with his secretary, Cajal heard shouting outside of his home, which they assumed to be coming from political demonstrators. The eighty-year-old Cajal slowly made his way up onto his balcony, overlooking a street that borders Retiro Park. As soon as he stepped outside, there were loud cheers; the mob turned out to be a group of university students who had heard that Cajal was ill. They skipped class to check on Cajal, the legendary founder of their school, despite the fact that he had not taught there for twelve years. Cajal was so overwhelmed with emotion that he could not speak. "I cannot ask anything more from life," he later told his closest disciple. Cajal deeply desired this form of acceptance, and yet it was difficult for him to accept demonstrations of affection.

Cajal's most explicit statements about the nature of the psyche come in his final book, *The World as Seen by an Eighty Year Old*. "As the modern psychologist has demonstrated," Cajal writes, "in each *I* there are various *egos* in intimate coexistence." His schema of the mind is similar to Freud's, with one significant difference. Although he agrees with Freud that the mind can be divided into smaller parts, Cajal rejects the Freudian unconscious. Cajal writes,

> Let us note that these secondary personalities are not unconscious, as a psychoanalyst might think, but rather subconscious and capable of easy evocation. They form as the rearguard of the current individual, but they are prepared to replace it as soon as it falters or becomes distracted.

Cajal worried that senility had rendered his dominant ego vulnerable to usurpation from rival psychic factions. If his "principal ego," which he calls "despotic and possessive," were to cede any control to attacks of subconscious suggestion, then his entire self-order would be destroyed.[15] These fears preoccupied the aging Cajal precisely when he began his diary.

In his diary, Cajal notes the interruption of many of his dreams due to intense attacks of emotional anguish. However, Cajal never inquires into the cause of these disturbances; in fact, any traumatic events suggested in his dreams are treated as lacking emotional significance. For example, when Cajal dreams about his university career, he cites the fact of his retirement, about which he was demonstrably upset, as though this chronological discrepancy empties the dream of any potential meaning. Similarly, when Cajal dreams that he is sitting next to his wife, he cites the fact that she is dead, as though this voids the symbolic weight of her imagined presence. The absence of feeling in response to her appearance in his dreams is astonishing; Cajal adored his wife, his partner for more than fifty years, and liked to echo his friends' observation that "half of Cajal is his wife."[16] After she died, Cajal altered his last will and testament to ensure that he would be buried next to her. Yet, even in his private diary, Cajal fails to acknowledge any wish to be with her again.

Throughout the diary, Cajal disqualifies his desires with a code word: "inconsistent." Cajal dreams about searching for sedatives in a strange pharmacy, and yet the insomniac admits neither his suffering nor his desire for peace. The crippled old man, who dreams of stealing grapes and running away with them, dismisses the dream as irrelevant on the ridiculous ground that grapes are no longer his favorite food. When he dreams about combat, he does not mention in his diary that he was once a soldier stationed at a battlefront hospital, where he witnessed the death of compatriots and almost perished himself. Cajal dismissed the dream as absurd because the scene did not include dead people. He remembers his past experience as a standard by which he can invalidate the dream, but he chooses not to explore that extremely painful interlude in his life.

Perhaps the most evocative material in the diary, which Cajal again fails to recognize, is a dream in which he drowns while holding his young daughter. Forty years earlier, Cajal lost a six-year-old daughter, Enriqueta, to bacterial disease. The most familiar biography of Cajal[17] maintains that he remained in his laboratory room while his wife screamed his name and beat on the door to alert him that their daughter was close to death. In this disputed account,[18] Cajal either did not hear or willfully ignored her cries. When he finally opened the door, he found his daughter's lifeless body in the arms of his wife. This dream proves that the death of his daughter had a profound and lasting effect on Cajal, even though he fails to admit as much.[19] Cajal's last secretary was a young girl named Enriqueta, who said that he treated her "like a father," whom he affectionately called "little one."[20]

Despite all of this charged material, there are few instances in the dream diary in which Cajal credits Freud's theory. The only wish that he openly admits is the desire to study botany. Cajal treats his dreams as though they were scientific propositions, beholden to the same rules of logic. As a professional scientist, his dominant ego thrived on will and disciplined reasoning; at his vulnerable age, any alternative traits were intolerable. There is no escaping the interpretation that despite the legitimate scientific, ideological, and political motivations behind Cajal's dream project, he was acting out a psychic conflict on the pages of his diary. Despite his stated objective to defeat Freud, for sixteen years Cajal was engaged in a secret dialogue with him. Despite insisting that the theories of psychoanalysis were "collective lies," he continually returned to conversation with a psychoanalyst.[21] Yet he was in denial of his psychic pain. Despite his visionary insights into the world of the infinitely small, Cajal failed to see larger meaning in his emotional condition. This blindness was a strategy that helped him to preserve the functioning of his scientific mind; these diaries are a testament to that cruel repression. The question is, How did such a mind become at once so great and so limited?

REFERENCES

1. Glick, "The Naked Science," 539.
2. See Rallo et al., "Introducción" to *Los sueños* (e.g., pp. 177, 195, and 287) for a thorough discussion of this theme, which helped me to form my ideas. The majority of the information about Cajal's decline comes from *Los sueños* and López Piñero, *Santiago Ramón y Cajal*.

3. Rallo et al., *Los sueños*, 36.
4. Manuel Barbeito Varvela, "Spanish and Spanish–American poetics and criticism," in *The Cambridge History of Literary Criticism: Volume IX, Twentieth-Century Historical, Philosophical and Psychological Perspectives*, ed. Crista Knellwolf and Christopher Norris (Cambridge, UK: Cambridge University Press, 2001), 351.
5. See Stahnisch and Nitsch, "Santiago Ramón y Cajal's Concept of Neuronal Plasticity."
6. L. Colucci-D'Amato, V. Bonavita, and U. di Porzio, "The End of the Central Dogma of Neurobiology: Stem Cells and Neurogenesis in Adult CNS," *Neurological Sciences* 27, no. 4 (September 2006), 266.
7. Rallo et al., "Introducción" to *Los sueños*, 40.
8. Cajal, *Advice*, 33.
9. "Madrid (From Our Regular Correspondent)," *Journal of the American Medical Association* 75, no. 6 (July 12, 1920).
10. Garcia López et al., "The Histological Slides."
11. Merchan et al., *Neurohistological Methods*, 14.
12. Rallo et al., "Introducción" to *Los sueños*, 99.
13. López-Muñoz et al., "The Neurobiological Interpretation of the Mental Function in the Work of Santiago Ramón y Cajal," 310.
14. Cajal, *Advice*, xv.
15. Cajal, *El mundo visto*, 181.
16. Cajal, *Recollections*, 272.
17. Alonso Buron, Francisco and Garcia Durán Muñoz, *Cajal: vida y obra*, 2nd ed. (Barcelona: Editorial Científico-Médico, 1983), 194.
18. Calvo, *Cajal*, 111; Luis Ramón y Cajal, "Cajal, as Seen by His Son," in *Proceedings of the Cajal Club 4* (1996), edited by Duane E. Haines, 76, http://cajalclub.org/sitebuildercontent/sitebuilderfiles/cajalbk4chap15cajalasseebyhisson.pdf; Juan Fernandez Santarén, "El problema de la neurogénesis," *Centro Virtual Cervantes*, http://cvc.cervantes.es/ciencia/cajal/cajal_recuerdos/introduccion_10.htm.
19. Cajal, *Recollections*, 380.
20. Rallo et al., "Introducción" to *Los sueños*, 261; Merchan et al., *The Neurohistological Methods*, 232.
21. Rallo et al., "Introducción," in *Los sueños*, 287.

CHAPTER 9

✧

"The Father of Modern Neuroscience" and His Father

Were Cajal ever to have participated in talk therapy, he undoubtedly would have spent most of his time talking about his father. From his father, Cajal claimed to inherit "everything that I am: belief in the sovereign will; faith in work; the conviction that a persevering and deliberate effort is capable of moulding and organizing everything, from the muscles to the brain."[1] Cajal's father was his first teacher and, he believed, his true master. Cajal's brother, Pedro Ramón y Cajal, also an important neuroanatomist, testified that only their father "glimpsed between the wild and chaotic undergrowth of the brain of Santiago, the light of a great intelligence capable of reaching brilliant victories in battles of intelligence."[2] His father was the dominating force throughout Cajal's development, and his complicated influence on Cajal was debated even by members of his own family. "They who feel that his father modeled him are mistaken," Cajal's son Luis said, "[Cajal] was a genius in spite of him."[3] The formation of Cajal's mind, including his attitude toward the psyche and his dreams, resulted from the unique dynamics of his relationship with his father, the role model for his repression.

Had he never had a son, history would have remembered Justo Ramón Casasús as the most remarkable man in his family. Born in Alto Aragón, a harsh and impoverished region in the mountains of northern Spain,[4] Ramón was the son of a farmer, whose land was parched and whose crops were meager. Because he was not the eldest son, Ramón was not in line for even this paltry inheritance. Aware of the utter lack of prospects, he left home at the age of twelve and apprenticed himself to a barber–surgeon in a nearby town, from whom he learned the medieval practice of cutting hair and letting blood. Barber–surgeons also tended to be more skillful in the art of dissection than doctors, who considered such manual labor to be undignified. Barber–surgeons were known as *romancistas*, a title that reflects their provincial status and lack of training in scholarly Latin.[5] However, Ramón's ambition was to study medicine. At age twenty-two, he traveled with his spare belongings to Barcelona, the ancient capital of Catalonia, a two-hundred-mile journey that he undertook on foot. Homeless, he managed to convince a local barber to let him work while earning a degree in surgery at the University of Barcelona. "From [my father]," Cajal writes, "I acquired also the beautiful ambition to be something worth while, and the determination to spare no sacrifice for the fulfilment of my aspirations, nor ever to deviate from the direct path on account of secondary motives or minor reasons."[6]

The royal road to Cajal's birthplace was a rugged bridle path.[7] Santiago Ramón y Cajal, the first child of Justo Ramón and Antonia Cajal Puente, was born in the tiny, isolated village of Petilla de Aragón, not much more than a pile of rocks on the side of a mountain, where his father served as the local surgeon. Ramón determined that his son would become a doctor even before his birth. It would be difficult to fault his intentions; to be a doctor meant guaranteed housing, a consistent salary, and an esteemed social status. His pursuit of a medical profession had lifted him from abject poverty into a more comfortable and less anxious life. However, his ambition and sacrifice did not stop there. "Don Justo," as he was respectfully called, continued to study medicine, eventually earning his doctorate. For a man born into such disadvantaged circumstances to elevate his status to such a degree was almost unimaginable. The six-year-old Cajal watched his father ride off to Madrid to achieve his dream. In the eyes of the son, the father was a hero; in the eyes of the father, the son could be molded in his image.

Don Justo saw himself as a natural pedagogue, a self-appointed authority who felt no compunction about correcting even those children who were not his own. When Cajal was four, his father started teaching him the basics of reading, writing, arithmetic, geography, physics, and even French. Their classroom was a cave that shepherds had abandoned. Cajal learned how to learn from his father, at a time and place where such early academic pursuits were extremely unusual. If Cajal were the son of another man, he might not have had more than an elementary education. Like most of Spain, especially the most rural areas, Alto Aragón was submerged in Catholicism, and although both father and son were baptized, they practiced a different religion, worshipping the wonders of science. When Cajal was eight years old, his father explained the natural laws predicting a solar eclipse, and the two of them marveled at the order of the universe while the rest of the villagers reacted with confusion and fear. If he were raised in a traditional environment, more consistent with the intellectual values of his neighbors, Cajal almost certainly would never have become a scientist.

In these ways, the influence of Cajal's father was progressive, providing a model of hard work and achievement and a foundation for knowledge and education. However, his example as a parent fell between the modern and the medieval. In many ways, Cajal's character differed from his father's, and this incongruence led to intense friction. Cajal preferred being alone to any social interaction, whereas his father maintained that success was a function of one's social and political role in the community. Facing less severe deprivation than his father had growing up, Cajal was less driven to overcome his surroundings. Whereas his father was gifted with an encyclopedic verbal memory, the key to his academic success, Cajal was a visual learner who struggled to retain words and recite texts. This difference was an early source of conflict; Cajal struggled to memorize Latin declensions, and only with this knowledge could he exceed the position of a romancista, a crucial achievement from his father's point of view.

This conflict was only amplified when, at the age of eight, Cajal became obsessed with drawing. Like many distractible students, he doodled in his books sketching epic battle scenes, holy saints, and armored heroes during class, and he was hopelessly tempted by the whiteness of walls, marking them with images, sometimes obscene. Whatever money he came upon, he spent on pencils and paper. He sketched everything in his sight: villagers, horses, carts, all slightly idealized, according to his juvenile worldview. For color, he devised a method of soaking the bindings of cigarette paper, extracting reds and blues. All of this subversive activity led him to spend even more time alone. "Translating my dreams onto paper," he writes, "with my pencil as a magic wand, I constructed a world according to my own fancy, containing all those etchings which nourished my dreams."[8] The first dream of Santiago Ramón y Cajal was to become a professional artist.

Cajal's father believed that the human mind was a machine designed to accumulate facts and to acquire knowledge. Through severe renunciation, he had been able to concentrate his intellectual efforts and achieve almost mythic success. Don Justo demanded that his son emulate the same utilitarian discipline. He banned works of fiction; only medical books were allowed in the house. To Cajal's father, every second that Cajal did not spend studying for his future career was not merely wasteful but also dangerous. Cajal's father took the position that if, after becoming a successful doctor, Cajal still wished to draw, then he would have plenty of time for that hobby. In the meantime, Cajal's father would confiscate and destroy any drawings and art materials he found.

Cajal's father was a tyrant who demanded ultimate obedience; any deviance was severely punished. In fact, Cajal's father tortured him, favoring such barbaric weapons as cudgels and tongs. A Spanish saying embodies the cruelty of this treatment: *La letra con sangre entra,* or "Knowledge comes with blood."[9] In response to the pain, Cajal learned to thicken his skin and to numb himself. Not only did he persist in his rebellious behavior but also rebellion became an expression of his art. To counteract Cajal's growing defiance, his father sent him away to a medical preparatory school, run by Jesuit fathers, whose dogmatic headmaster had a reputation for "breaking colts."[10] Cajal's teachers beat, imprisoned, and starved him for his insubordination and his failure to learn Latin. Don Justo was approximately his son's age when he left home, and thus he was unsympathetic to the boy's hardships, which must have been nothing compared to those he had faced growing up. When, after Cajal and his brother ran away from home, their father found them sleeping in a cave, he shook them awake, beat them, tied their arms together, and publicly humiliated them by dragging them through the streets of town. Cajal assimilated these abusive experiences into his worldview by adopting the philosophy that pain is a necessary stimulant to creativity.

Cajal's father treated Cajal's artistic impulses as symptoms of a psychological disease, which he tried time and again to eradicate. When a traveling painter came to town to whitewash the walls of the church, Don Justo asked this eminent art critic to judge whether his son had any talent. Because Don Justo was an important figure, the painter delivered the expected verdict: The eleven-year-old boy's work was completely without merit. Cajal's hopes were destroyed, and he never again entertained the idea of being a professional artist. For this, history probably owes Don Justo begrudging thanks. Although Cajal was undeniably talented for his age, as his extant canvasses demonstrate, he would have likely become, by his own admission, a second-rate Romantic painter. Not only would he have plummeted in the social hierarchy, as his father feared, but also the world would have lost a uniquely creative scientist, whose mind always was inspired by visual and aesthetic sensitivities. Throughout his adolescence, Cajal continued to draw in secret, especially inspired by scenes of natural beauty. His father, angry that he neglected his studies, removed Cajal for a year from school and apprenticed him to a cobbler. However, Cajal thrived, despite the deprivation, embracing the trade and befriending the clientele. He even managed to smuggle in drawing materials, which his father had insisted would be forbidden. Despite his father's punishments, no matter what his circumstances, Cajal's love of drawing was never extinguished.

Don Justo never stopped trying to draw his son into medicine. One night, when Cajal was sixteen years old, his father secretly led him into a local graveyard, handing the boy a shovel and instructing him in hushed tones to dig up the corpse, which they carried back to the family's barn. There, under the light of gas lamps, Don Justo deftly demonstrated the art of dissection, carving out muscle and bone, explaining the intricacies of the body in exacting detail, surprising Cajal by extolling the virtues of direct observation and admitting the limitations of studying texts. Don Justo valorized the role of the surgeon, glorifying the special caliber of vision that is necessary to guide the scalpel through opaque territories. Cajal was utterly astounded; in dead bodies, he saw the mechanisms of life revealed. He suddenly realized that human beings were the most beautiful of all the objects in nature.

The experience was unforgettable. From this point on, anatomy was Cajal's favorite subject, both in his schoolwork and in his art. Most profoundly, anatomy represented a hesitant reconciliation between Cajal and his father; if they could connect at all, it would be through the medium of anatomy. Although Cajal's father finally triumphed in his quest to direct his son toward medical studies, Cajal, as always, approached the discipline on his own terms. As Pedro later articulated in his brother's eulogy, Cajal "entered the castle of Science through the door of Art."[11] "There can be no doubt that only artists are attracted to science," Cajal told an interviewer, "I owe what I am today to boyhood artistic hobbies, which my father opposed fiercely."[12]

When Cajal enrolled in medical school, Don Justo accompanied his son to the provincial capital of Zaragoza and placed him under the supervision of a trusted friend. Then, Don Justo moved the family to Zaragoza so that he could be closer to his son and ensure the rectitude of his course. Don Justo had friends who were professors at the university, and soon he became a temporary instructor in anatomy. According to the Spanish tradition, Cajal's professors referred to him by his father's name: "Ramón." Cajal physically resembled Don Justo to such an extent that people mistook him for his father. However, when Cajal's father was in medical school, he applied all of his mental resources toward his studies while struggling to earn a living. On the other hand, while Cajal excelled in anatomy and pathology, he neglected the work for his other courses, choosing instead to spend time exploring the landscape and drawing.

After Cajal's graduation, Don Justo sensed momentum and urged his son to apply immediately for a doctorate, matching his own achievement.

When Cajal was ordered to Cuba, his father pleaded with him not to go. Don Justo even procured a letter of recommendation from one of his influential friends to steer his son toward a more favorable deployment, away from the dangers of the jungle. Cajal never exercised this privilege, choosing romantic adventure over prudence, and, as a result, fell prey to precisely the perils that his father augured. Despite traveling thousands of miles across the ocean against Don Justo's wishes, Cajal's hopes for a long-sought separation were dashed, and he was forced to again submit to his father's guidance and care.

When he returned home, Cajal was reliant on his father while he convalesced. It was his father who arranged for his job at the Anatomical Museum at the University of Zaragoza; for three years, Cajal worked as an auxiliary professor, assisting Don Justo in the dissection room, the most natural atmosphere, where Cajal enjoyed learning from his father, just as he had in the cave. In fact, Don Justo finally recognized the value of his son's talent, and the two embarked on the creation of an anatomical atlas, which Cajal illustrated. However, their conflict persisted, stemming from the tension between Don Justo's insistence on absolute conformity and Cajal's desire for self-expression. One day, after Cajal refused his father's request for assistance with an obstetrical procedure, a fierce argument resulted in Cajal leaving the house for days.[13] The tension between clinical practice, Don Justo's vocation, and biological research, the devotion of his son, was a continuous source of family strife.[14]

While Cajal earned his doctorate, inspiring his father's pride, he also discovered histology, which became his own passion and opened a path toward independence. Don Justo wanted his son to participate in *oposiciones*; Cajal would have preferred first to deepen his study of microscopic technique, an unconventional discipline not practiced by most anatomists of his father's generation. "My aspirations to an academic appointment," Cajal admits, "were prompted continually by my father rather than felt spontaneously."[15] The intense pressures of oposiciones appear in anxiety dreams decades later; the competitive examinations, after all, would determine lifetime appointments. Cajal writes that he felt his failure "most keenly because of the disappointment and disillusion which it was going to cause my father and teacher."[16] A few months later, Cajal experienced those symptoms that he identified as tubercular. In any person, hypochondriasis is a complex disorder; in the son of a doctor, obsession with serious illness assumes an even greater psychological significance.

Cajal had to cope with a profound need for a father who both tried to destroy him and saved his life. If Don Justo were not an educated man of medicine, he might not have sent his son for hydrotherapy, the leading cure of the day. At Panticosa, Cajal refused the advice of all of the doctors, as though he were denying substitutes for his father, whose prescriptions he felt had wounded him throughout his life. When Cajal returned, Don Justo tried to force him into the perceived safety of a clinical practice by arranging for an job for his son in a rural town. This represented a recapitulation of Don Justo's own career as country doctor. Cajal briefly consented before officially refusing the offer. In 1883, at the age of thirty-two, Cajal finally won an oposicion that earned him the appointment to Valencia. When he finally moved away from his father, the separation was definitive. Cajal never returned to Zaragoza, where his family lived, even when he had the opportunity.

Probably the final time that Cajal saw his father was in 1892. Cajal was on his way to his new appointment in Madrid when he stopped in Zaragoza to visit his ailing mother. While there, he learned that his father, by then an old man, had impregnated a peasant girl from the town where he served as the parish doctor and had abandoned his wife. Cajal adored his mother; in the midst of his father's tyranny, she was his only savior. She had secreted novels to him, despite his father's ban, and beseeched his father to put an end to the boy's cruel treatment at the Jesuit school until he finally relented. Antonia Cajal died in 1898. Identifying as a Catholic, Don Justo believed that he needed to marry the girl whom he had impregnated and to raise the child in a family. Cajal's siblings forgave their father; his sisters eventually moved in with him, and even Pedro, who was practicing medicine in Zaragoza just like his father, eventually resumed contact. Cajal never spoke to his father again.[17]

REFERENCES

1. Cajal, *Recollections*, 4.
2. Pedro Ramón y Cajal, "La juventud de Cajal contada por su hermano Don Pedro," in *La psicología de las artistas*, 3rd edition (Madrid: Espasa Calpe, S.A., 1972), 19.
3. Ramón y Cajal, "Cajal, As Seen by His Son," 73.
4. López Piñero, *Santiago Ramón y Cajal*, 103.
5. Manuel A. Fuentes, *Lima: Or Sketches of the Capital of Peru, Historical, Statestical, Administrative, Commercial, and Moral* (Paris: Firman Didot, Brothers, Sons & Co., 1866), 164.
6. Cajal, *Recollections*, 4-5.
7. Cajal, *Recollections*, 9.
8. Cajal, *Recollections*, 36.
9. Laura Otis, "Introduction," in *Vacation Stories*, ix.
10. Cajal, *Recollections*, 14.
11. Pedro Ramón y Cajal, "La juventud de Cajal," 28.

12. Javier DeFelipe, *Cajal's Butterflies of the Soul*, title page.
13. "Cajal, As Seen By His Son, by Luis Ramón y Cajal," in *Proceedings of the Cajal Club* 4 (1996), 73.
14. Calvo Roy, *Cajal*, 146; Muñoz and Burón, *Cajal*, 253.
15. Cajal, *Recollections*, 248.
16. Cajal, *Recollections*, 255.
17. Antonio Calvo Roy, *Cajal: Triunfar a Toda Costa* (Madrid: Alianza Editorial, 2007), 146.

CHAPTER 10

✧

The Dream Diary's Strange Fate

Despite the blatant trauma his father's treatment caused him, Cajal never addresses the relationship in his diary, even when his dreams present the opportunity. For example, after a dream about delivering a baby, Cajal recalls that he used to help his father in obstetrics, but he does not mention any of the attendant disputes. In another dream, Cajal is anxious because he has forgotten the names of some bones in the hand, and he recites the names of the bones as soon as he awakens, "from memory with no mistakes." Fifty years later, he is proud to demonstrate his capacity for memorization. Although he mentions that his father taught him anatomy at a young age, Cajal does not recall any other history, even though memorization was a unique source of conflict between them. Finally, after a dream about hiding a checkbook in the sand, Cajal notes that during his childhood, he used to hide precious objects, such as drawings, among the rocks—a memory that is repeated in his autobiography. However, although the image of saving his artwork from being eradicated by his father is a perfect symbol for Cajal's deep and painful struggle, Cajal does not mention any of his emotions from that time at all.

It becomes clear from reading the dream diary that Cajal treats his dreams in the same way that his father treated him when Cajal was a child. The dominant traits with which Cajal identifies, such as effort, will, and perseverance, formed his professional ego, reinforced by decades of disciplined scientific work. Cajal displays no tolerance for the significance of dreams; he repeatedly dismisses them, calling them absurd, an echo of his father's belittling of his own artistic impulse. "The critical self," the autocratic force that threatens the direct communication of a dream report, was embodied by his father.

Despite his attempts to circumvent his father's influence, Cajal continued to emulate Don Justo's qualities, among which repression was central,
and thus he unwittingly mimicked his father's personality. Cajal's "senile
ego" suffered from the accumulation of such intensely complicated feelings toward his father, which the force of his father's example prevented
him from expressing. The dream diary, which may have started out as a
scientific project, became an artifact of this personal struggle, implying
a psychic life that Cajal tries to keep from the text itself. Perhaps Cajal
realized that his new book would fail to disprove Freud and that he had no
alternative theory to offer, and so he subjected the work to the same rea-
sonable censorship as his earlier attempts at psychological explanation.
Although his choice not to publish seems obvious and consistent with his
intellectual values, his subsequent decision about the fate of the manuscript is surprising and betrays a deeper emotional ambivalence.

Cajal's last will and testament[1] bequeathed his scientific materials, such
as microscopes and histological preparations, to his disciples at the Cajal
Institute, and he left his personal belongings, such as books and awards,
to his family. Two years after Cajal's death, in July 1936, the Spanish Civil
War erupted, and Madrid was besieged for almost three years. While many
of Cajal's students died, were exiled, or fled, two of his closest disciples,
Fernando de Castro and Jorge Francisco Tello, stayed to defend the Cajal
Institute and guard their master's archives.[2] After the war, Cajal's family
agreed to store their property at the Cajal Institute, in the hopes of creating a museum dedicated to his legacy. The archives of Santiago Ramón
y Cajal contain more than thirty thousand items,[3] including childhood
drawings, travel photographs, thousands of scientific drawings on scraps
of paper and in sketchbooks, as well as histological slides of brain tissue
still gummy to the touch. All of these artifacts currently are stored in a
small temperature- and humidity-controlled meeting room on the same
hall as the laboratories at the Cajal Institute.[4] The mysterious dream book
of Cajal is not among the two thousand handwritten manuscripts there;[5]
scholars generally assumed that the unpublished work was lost during the
Spanish Civil War.[6]

In fact, Cajal's unfinished dream book was not a formal manuscript but,
rather, a collection of loose sheets of used paper and notes in the margins
of newspapers and magazines.[7] Cajal did not publish the work, but neither
did he consider the attempt to be such a failure that the pages were not
valuable. He did not give the diary to his family or closest disciples. Just
before he died, Cajal surreptitiously handed over this material to a man
named José Germain Cebrían,[8] who had studied medicine under Cajal at
the University of Madrid. In a class taught by Gonzalo Rodríguez Lafora,
one of Cajal's main students, Germain studied neuropsychiatry, in which

he decided to specialize. In 1923, after earning his doctorate, Germain studied abroad, having been awarded a grant by the national organization that Cajal headed. In Geneva, Germain encountered psychoanalysis, toward which he developed a positive attitude.

When he returned to Spain, Germain worked at Lafora's Neuropsychiatry Sanatorium, part of Cajal's inner circle, and also served as the chief editor of the *Neurobiology Archives*. In Cajal's mind, Germain was an outstanding and well-rounded student, representing the best of the next generation of Spanish scientists: knowledgeable about contemporary psychology but respectful of his neurobiological school. Germain's autobiography recounts his deep respect for Cajal and a desire to venerate his legacy. There is no record of Cajal's instructions to Germain; however, by giving his dreams to such a figure, Cajal might have been hoping to ensure the future relevance of his ideas and to counteract his school's descent into obscurity, which he attributed to the spread of Freud's doctrines. Cajal could not have known how active Germain would become in the promotion of psychoanalysis.

At some point, Germain dutifully typed up the scattered diary into a proper manuscript, although Cajal's calligraphy often was illegible, including numerous errors, deletions, and blank spaces. When the Spanish Civil War broke out, like many intellectuals, Germain fled the country; he must have carried this secret manuscript with him for years. Germain spent time in Switzerland before traveling to Paris, where he became one of the few Spaniards at that time to undergo psychoanalysis, with Charles Odier, a follower of Freud and one of the founders of the Paris Psychoanalytic Society. In 1948, Germain was responsible for reorganizing and revising the collected works of Freud for Biblioteca, whose introduction he probably wrote himself.[9] Germain was working toward publishing Cajal's dreams when he decided to send the papers to a man named José Rallo, a younger Spanish psychologist. "As a psychoanalyst and having published works about dreams," Germain wrote to Rallo, "you are in a better position" to present them. The original dreams were ruined by a flood in Rallo's basement; Germain's manuscript version, ninety-six sheets, was recovered mysteriously in 2013. In Cajal's failed attempt to disprove Freud, the authors, three psychoanalysts, saw an implicit confirmation of psychoanalytic theory.[10]

In November 2014, the book *Los sueños de Santiago Ramón y Cajal* appeared in Spain.[11] The publication date is crucially significant; exactly eighty years after Cajal's death, his family's copyright expired and the intellectual property entered the public domain. The book's publisher is Biblioteca Nueva, the same Spanish press famous for producing the first complete works of Sigmund Freud during Cajal's lifetime.[12] The book's introduction,[13] a tremendously valuable resource, presents a psychoanalytic interpretation of Cajal's dreams, with discussions of classic themes such as infantile sexuality, the Oedipal complex, and libido. The authors' hypothesis is that, in the diary, Cajal transferred his ambivalent feelings toward his dead father onto the imaginary figure of Freud. Without a doubt, there is considerable irony, and even indignity, in the fact that, after his vigorous attempts to combat and negate Freudian theory, his work received the hated psychoanalytic treatment by Spanish disciples of Freud.

Cajal's manuscript, transcribed by José Germain Cebrían and reproduced in *Los sueños de Santiago Ramón y Cajal*, contains one hundred and three dreams. Almost all of the dreams are Cajal's own, with a few reported to him by his secretary and one by one of his granddaughters. Some of the entries are titled or dated, but most of them are not. There are many vivid, fascinating, and occasionally delightful entries. In one dream, Cajal's scalp is removed, and he feels that his brain is falling out. In another dream, the distinguished Nobel Laureate experiences the common fear that his pants fall down in public. One night, the champion of neuron theory dreams about having to explain the theory to an arena full of bullfighting fanatics who are also devout spiritualists. However, in an altered state of consciousness, the staunch empiricist also argues that the self is an invisible energy, like a god. Perhaps most revealingly, among the incessant dismissals of potential desires, Cajal admits a true and earnest wish: He would like to live long enough to "bring to light my observations about dreams." After eighty years, the pressures of Cajal's life were debilitating him, draining his psyche. "He who has consecrated a good part of his life to an order of intellectual activity," Cajal writes about himself in *The World as Seen*, "feels in his brain the silent fluttering of neglected regions."[14] What follows are the stirring, nearly incomprehensible whispers of this catharsis that never was.

REFERENCES

1. http://www.santiagoramonycajal.com.
2. Juan A. de Carlos and María Pedraza, "Santiago Ramón y Cajal: The Cajal Institute and the Spanish Histological School," *Anatomical Record* 297 (August 14, 2014), 1797, doi:10.1002/ar.23019.
3. Pablo Garcia-Lopez, Virginia Garcia Marin, and Miguel Freire, "The Histological Slides and Drawings of Cajal," *Frontiers in Neuroanatomy* 4 (March 10, 2010), doi:10.3389/neuro.05.009.2010.
4. Personal visit to the Cajal Legacy in March 2015.
5. Garcia-Lopez et al., "The Histological Slides."

6. Rallo et al., *Los sueños*, 13; Ramón y Cajal, "Santiago Ramón y Cajal y la hipnosis."

7. Rallo et al., "Introducción" to *Los sueños*.

8. Rallo et al., "Introducción" to *Los sueños*, 15–20; Fernanda Monasterio, "Las obras de José Germain," *Papeles de psicólogo*, nos. 28 and 29 (February 1982), http://www. papelesdelpsicologo.es/vernumero.asp?id=315; Juan Antonio Mora, "Semblanza Biográfica del Dr. D. José Germain Cebrián," *General de Colegios Oficiales de Psicólogos*, no. 70 (June 1998), http://www.cop.es/infocop/vernumeroCOP.asp?id=991.

9. Rallo et al., "Introducción" to *Los sueños*, 23.

10. Rallo et al., "Introducción" to *Los sueños*, 23.

11. Rallo et al., "Introducción" to *Los sueños*.

12. Glick, "The Naked Science," 108.

13. Rallo et al., "Introducción" to *Los sueños*, 1–365.

14. Cajal, *El mundo visto*, 181.

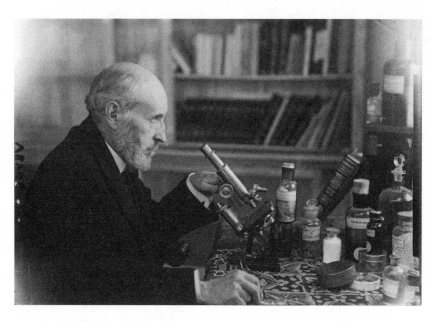

Figure 1 The elderly Cajal at the microscope.
Source: Courtesy Cajal Legacy, Instituto Cajal (CSIC), Madrid.

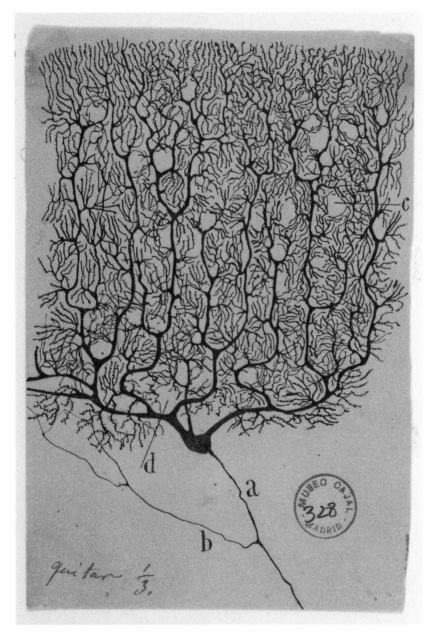

Figure 2 Human Purkinje cell in the human cerebellum, 1899–1904. Reproduced in *Butterflies of the Soul* (DeFelipe), Figure F-5.

Source: Courtesy Cajal Legacy, Instituto Cajal (CSIC), Madrid.

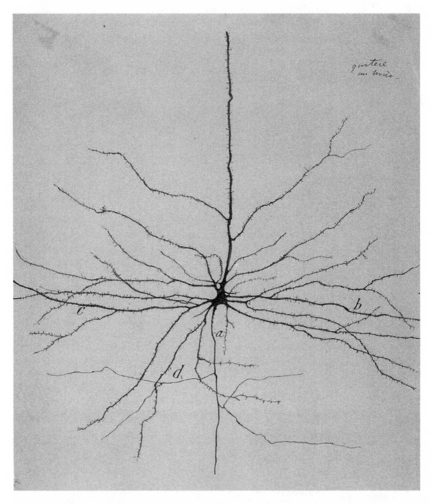

Figure 3 Pyramidal cell of the human motor cortex, 1899. Reproduced in "The dendritic spine story: an intriguing process of discovery" (DeFelipe), Figure 5.
Source: Courtesy Cajal Legacy, Instituto Cajal (CSIC), Madrid.

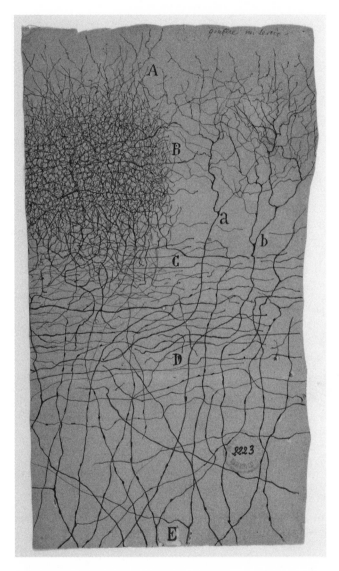

Figure 4 Sensory plexus of the human cerebral cortex, 1899. Reproduced in *Butterflies of the Soul* (DeFelipe), Figure 31.
Source: Courtesy Cajal Legacy, Instituto Cajal (CSIC), Madrid.

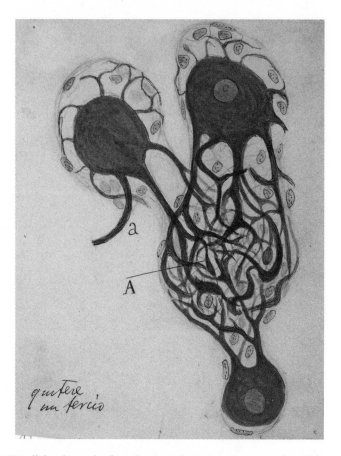

Figure 5 Tricellular glomerulus from the sympathetic nervous system of an adult man, 1905. Reproduced in *Butterflies of the Soul* (DeFelipe), Figure 40.
Source: Courtesy Cajal Legacy, Instituto Cajal (CSIC), Madrid.

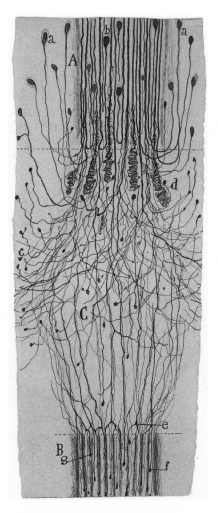

Figure 6 Schematic drawing showing the regeneration of a cut nerve, 1905. Reproduced in "Sesquicentenary of the Birthday of Santiago Ramón y Cajal" (DeFelipe), Figure 6.
Source: Courtesy Cajal Legacy, Instituto Cajal (CSIC), Madrid.

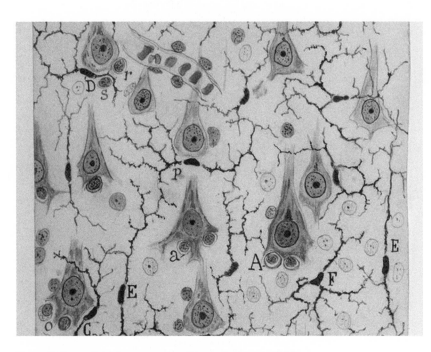

Figure 7 Neuroglia in the gray matter of the cerebral cortex, 1920.
Source: Courtesy Cajal Legacy, Instituto Cajal (CSIC), Madrid.

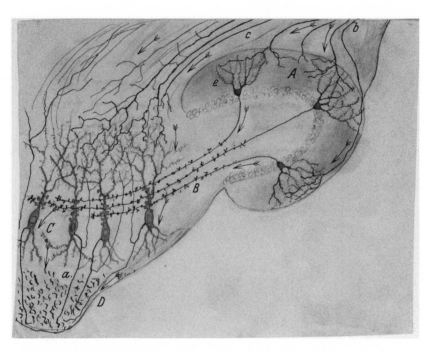

Figure 8 Schematic drawing of the connection between fascia dentata and Ammon's horn.
Source: Courtesy Cajal Legacy, Instituto Cajal (CSIC), Madrid.

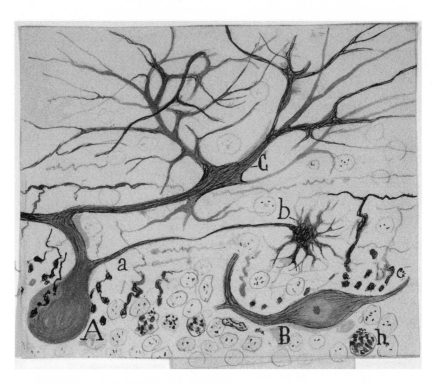

Figure 9 Purkinje cells in a case of dementia precox, 1926.
Source: Courtesy Cajal Legacy, Instituto Cajal (CSIC), Madrid.

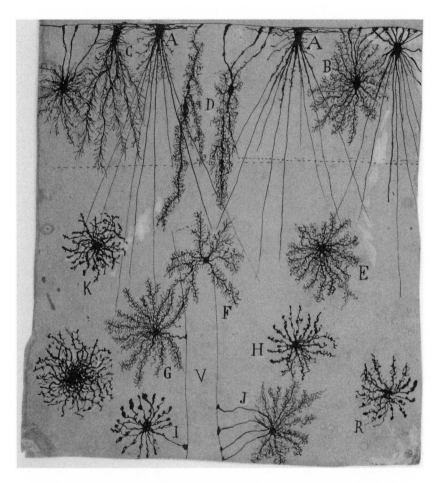

Figure 10 Neuroglia in the cerebrum of a two-month-old child. Reproduced in *Butterflies of the Soul* (DeFelipe), Figure F-33.
Source: Courtesy Cajal Legacy, Instituto Cajal (CSIC), Madrid.

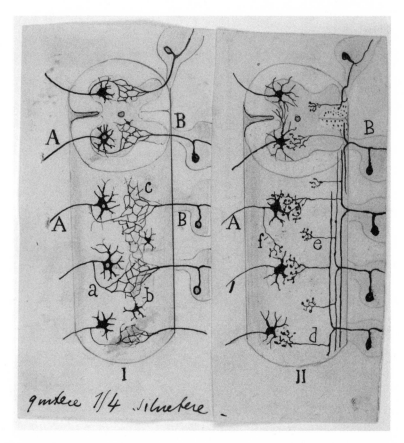

Figure 11 The differences between the neuron and reticular theories regarding the sensory-motor connections of the spinal cord, with Cajal's scheme on the left (I) and Golgi's on the right (II). Reproduced in *Butterflies of the Soul* (DeFelipe), Figure F-34.
Source: Courtesy Cajal Institute, CSIC. Madrid, Spain.

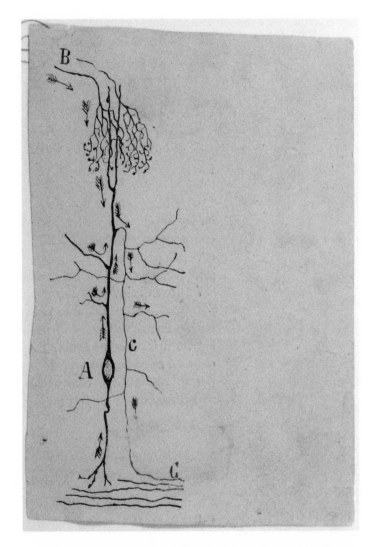

Figure 12 The flow of electric current from cells in the retina to the optic lobe of a sparrow, illustrating the concept of dynamic polarity. Reproduced in *Cajal's Butterflies of the Soul* (DeFelipe), Figure F-36.

Source: Courtesy Cajal Legacy, Instituto Cajal (CSIC), Madrid.

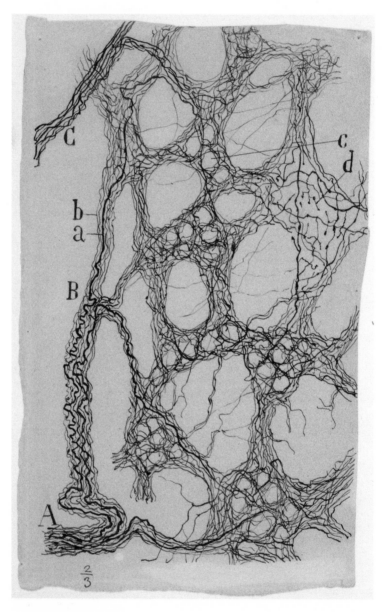

Figure 13 Auerbach plexus and ganglia of a mouse, 1893. Reproduced in *Cajal's Butterflies of the Soul* (DeFelipe), Figure 20.
Source: Courtesy Cajal Legacy, Instituto Cajal (CSIC), Madrid.

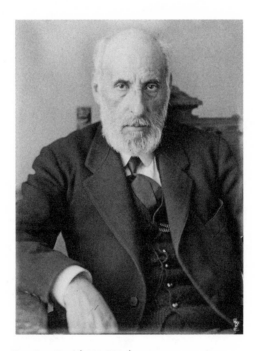

Figure 14 Santiago Ramón y Cajal (1852–1934).
Source: Courtesy Cajal Legacy, Instituto Cajal (CSIC), Madrid.

PART 2

The Dream Diary
of Santiago Ramón y Cajal

CHAPTER 11

৩৬৩

The Dreams of Cajal

Original By Santiago Ramón y Cajal
Transcribed by José Germain Cebrián
Reproduced by José Rallo Romero
Translated into English by Benjamin Ehrlich

✳✳✳ = cross-out
[-----] = blank space

FREUD THEORY

Every dream is the ✳✳✳ fulfillment of a desire repressed by the conscience.
    Every dream is the fulfillment of an infantile desire.
    Dreams have an egotistical source, almost always of sexual origin even
if something else appears. They were burdened much of childhood when
the censor was not operating and [-----].

— The evocative cause pertains to the day on which one dreams.
— One does not reason in a dream, that which appears to be reasoning is
    reproduction of a mental image. Delage is critical and says that a dream
    is rarely a fulfillment of repressed desire.

Taken from Delage, Inst. Psych., 1915

DREAM (5 A.M.) APRIL 1918

I am delivering a speech before a popular auditorium. Atheneum. I talk ✳✳✳ about the neuron theory. Passion, eloquence while speaking about how the form was discovered and recounting the miracles of the Golgi and Ehrlich methods. I forget nothing. But I grow tired of talking and a moment comes when I ask myself am I not dreaming? I awaken.

It explains the theory of disuse. I have not talked about of this for a long time. Athaeneum lecture reminiscence. I have no desire to address this subject excessively treated in books. No such nonsense. That which one [-----] is [-----] from memory. There is no creation, rather it comes from some quotation.

THOUGHTS THAT OCCURRED IN FANTASIES

16 of May 1918

The art of instincts is nothing but the sum of instincts ^{ancestor animals}/ which man remembers vaguely from the past and which he perfects and improves. This shows that intellectual acts are forgotten instinctual resources. (Critic: Man has not gone through the insect series, and others that offer similar capacities. The savage is ignorant of them.)

Philosophy provides ethnographic characteristics, but not qualities of the truth. It represents the way the Saxon, the German, the Latin X value the history of the world and its profound reality. Dreams are philosophical systems realized. Here the idea of Freud's dream theory is applied well.

(These ideas are ideas from fantasy conversations, May 1918)

COMMON DREAM

10 of May 1918

I attend a diplomatic soiree and as I am leaving my pants fall down (Is it desire?).

I take a walk by the bay and I fall into the water with one of my little daughters in my arms. I fight the waves, I am almost drowning, still touching the seawall (Santander?). The nightmare awakens me.

DREAM AND SOME EXPLANATION (CHILDHOOD)

18 of May 1918

Out of curiosity I entered an orchard by jumping the wall. While walking I notice that there were people, women hanging clothes, and without flinching I run underneath the wall and in a place [------] where there were hanging clothes I get ready to leave and I leave. When I come out I meet a woman who freezes a little bit when she recognizes an old man. I apologize ✶✶✶ telling her that having leaned over the edge my glasses had fallen and I had taken the liberty of going down to retrieve them, so that she would not think something else. The woman accepted the excuse and let me leave.

Note: The excuse was an instantaneous and new invention for my own orchard as I never saw that other one, it had walls on the other side carved out of a hill and extremely high, at least as high as a house. We were in winter. There was no fruit.

Are childhood memories the preferred image? But there are new things as well.

Now dreams are usually about talking, giving classes or lectures on scientific, philosophical, or political themes. More infrequently about my discoveries. The fact is that I neither have the opportunity to speak (silence cure) nor to discuss them. Almost every day I leave with a headache from so much talking. The silence cure does not work for me, then.

It is peculiar that this talking in dreams does not bother me as much as conversation while awake.

DREAM

On Sunday September 6 of 1918 Swiss and Germans were aiming into my orchard and the whole time we had to constantly ask them to let us pass so we could go down to the garden. Then precisely on that night I dream that a strange woman in a park or garden was entertaining herself by shooting at me through some trees with a toy pistol and I was moving my head to avoid being hit.

This game awakens me.

DREAMS

The fact that the most emotional and fatiguing events of the day are not an influence is proven by these two very repetitive cases (by analogy).

1. I dream that I speak in front of students about mossy fibers and about the fact that no one knows where they come from.
2. The evening until 8:30 was spent on an automobile drive to the Santillana dam, Manzanares and its castle.
3. When I lie down in bed I read the speech by Rodriguez Marín about Magdalene ([-----]).

What could have evoked that from the cerebellum? A work completed under my direction in my Laboratory by a Canadian, Norton Crarigie who two days earlier submitted it to me for publication.

Countless times in *opposiciones*, lectures and emotional ceremonies, I dreamt about ordinary things, having gone to bed almost feverish and full of the day's excitements and concerns.

DREAM

That a committee of professors comes to my house to beg me to give a course on the Histology of the nervous system, or to reinstate me in a new committee chair, after being retired. That I refuse citing the poor state of my health.

Some of this was unofficial; but I did not want it. So much so that those final months, overwhelmed by arteriosclerosis and deafness, I had my assistants teaching classes. Neither did I want to give a farewell lecture. I was afraid of the warmth of the public, the expectation and the emotion which in my state would only be damaging to me, since I have only sad memories from the final classes. For the same reasons I did not attend Academies, nor theaters and I have suspended my tertulia conversations at the Suizo.

DREAM

I walk past a cathedral under construction. The chapels are being used to grow cabbage and chard. The custodian's chickens wander here and there. Some columns are completely covered with lichen. Nearby there is [-----] of a dirty and squalid café where 203 construction workers play dominoes. I get ready to eat the swill that they serve me. It appears to me that I am a student who has come to Madrid with little money accompanied by a friend.

Recurring dream.

Causes, perhaps having read about the impossibility of finishing the Church of Jesus.

Underlying: the [-----] ruins of the cathedral and of the Basilica Atocha.

ACOUSTIC DREAM

Teaching classes. There is perfect logic and good memory for words and concepts. The inconsistency lies in the fact that either the material is not familiar to us or we believe we are professors without being one and our audience is scarce or great. None of these things have to do with the libido. One of my final lessons is on the normal and pathological anatomy of the ear and examines deafness and I continue with my class until I realize that I am not a professor, and that it is absurd that I gave a lecture.

(Here the influence of habit loads nerve cells with [-----] fluid. They are established pathways, mnemonic phenomena and conditions that did not want to die, that reveal themselves.

That there is a bit of this one sees in people who because of the state of their health cannot speak; and as soon as they have the opportunity they are inexhaustible (drunkenness of words).

MORNING DREAM

12 December 1926

After lecturing in the seminar room about who knows which philosoph-ical topics. I find myself among friends. The issue of what constitutes the elements of human nature arises, I do not know how. Without letting anyone else speak in an authoratative tone and capturing the attention of my listeners—all friends and colleagues—(I hear myself proclaim-ing vehemently), I declare that the [------] doctrines of the unity of the human individual is an illusion, that within us in reality there are four men:

1. *The gangue man*, the cellular cadaver, the connective tissue, bone ✳✳✳, intercellular materials X. It is the filler of life. Stature strength is the façade and the filler of the building.
2. *The glandular and sympathetic man*, that is to say, the colllection of internal and external secretory organs, coordinated by the ✳✳✳ sym-pathetic ganglia governing vegetative life and whose influence higher individuals (emotional, synaesthetic) and the gangue man must endure.
3. *The pneumonic and conscious man*, that is to say, the cerebral nervous system, the registry where sensory residues are stored. It is united by the senses to the exterior world and to the higher self by certain

cerebral pathways. This self can be conscious (sensation, perception) however it generally remains in a state of storage for primary ideals (the unconscious of many authors). It produces the reflexive and intuitive moment. The higher self is that active, imperious, conscious impulse, the selector that consults the files of the cerebral library, that [-----] the pathways, chooses useful and deliberate reactions; attends to sensation, or does not; represses reflexes, moderates instincts and forges ideas and theories changing the sensory material of the mind. This self *is the critical self,* that sees but is not seen, that in the dream state (hallucinatory orgy of the 2nd self, fed up with contradictions says: Enough; all of this is an illusion, let us awaken. Believing that a representation is the self is like thinking that a photographic lens depicts itself. Maybe if there were a mirror in front. But in man the self has no mirror. The self is absolutely inaccessible. That which we take for a mirror, consciousness, only shows us the product of the [-----] selection thought to be the object but what is thought to be the object is not what we think, but rather yet another part of our images about which one thinks . . .

The self is an energy, an invisible pull like a god . . .
Here I awaken.

DREAM

12th of December 1926

Theft in my laboratory. Someone who was watching for the moment when I left for the night and was alone, he came out to the balconies.

He had to climb up the balcony, he broke open a drawer and stole 1 to 2 pesetas. I told this to some friends.

Preceding elements. The doorman warning that I must not leave money there, because they could climb up the balcony and steal it. This warning was 30 or 40 days before (Freud's desire?) Libido?

Reality. The robbery did not happen. It was all imagined. It was the echo of a piece of advice.

Immediately after I dream that people were asking dean Calleja to borrow 2,000 pts. for a professor who had previously been told that his baldness could be cured. Calleja loaned them the money and his baldness was not cured. The dream is harmless.

Real elements: 25 years ago the newly appointed Chacón asked him for money and returned it.

In a barbershop they told me that N. a friend of mine who is extremely bald, for 25 years, was in the process of treatment. To which I replied that if the drug could cure a man as bald as that it should be certified. But N. was not cured.

A discussion followed about the thoughtless confabulation of newspapers, and the indifference of the health authorities who seem not to care when people are robbed by certain businessmen and taken in by their claims, and every terminal patient is persuaded to buy what they say is good.

DREAM OF THE PRINTING HOUSE

I find myself at a printer correcting proofs of a book about regeneration. I discover that there are many letters missing, that prepositions are missing, and that syllables have run over from one line to the next. I am shocked and ashamed by all these errors.

Inconsistencies. I am not correcting proofs of a book in the process of being printed, but rather of a book that is printed and already for sale, and also translated into English. My corrections are pointless, then. Moreover the book, of which I do not wish to make a new edition, was printed 12 years ago. I awaken.

Strong headache due to the suffocating heat upon checking the already inevitable errors. I am in Jaca.

This cannot be explained by Freud.

There is nothing here but a reminiscence of a previous event with distortions.

I imagine that I am at Pueyo's press, where the book was not made. New inconsistency.

DREAM

23 of April 1927

In who knows what embassy [-----] I ask [-----] obligingly and in French for a grant from the English government for having helped Tagore the Indian poet translate the Vedas into English.

Absurd: I hardly know the Vedas. I am completely ignorant of Sanskrit. I do not know the Indian poet nor do I know if he has attempted to translate anything. I detest poetry, even myth except for the Odyssey and the Iliad.

Even if all else were true it is inconceivable that I would dare ask for money from the English government instead of from the person to whom I had lent the service.

Indirect cause: immediate: having read an article the night before in La Esfera in which Tagore is discussed on the occasion of his impressions of Europe.

Remote cause: having read some translation of Tagore's poetry which was awarded the Nobel and many years ago having read some translated passage of the Mahabarata Vedas.

DREAM

10 of May 1927

Long trip with several naturalists in search of ants. Study of the barbarous [-----] eager to see if it is agricultural. Ravenous thirst. The snack is made and we have nothing but wine. I want to drink water. A pastor comes with a jar full of muddy water. He tells me that it has been collected in a pool frequented by cattle. Reluctance to drink it and therefore more thirst.

The thirst awakens me and I drink water (4 in the morning).

Incidental cause: having seen harvester ants in Boubier, "Le communisme chez les insectes," Paris, 1926.

Underlying cause: my studies about ants and the heat of the sun for me in May. This provided the combined sensory details.

DREAM

Today, 9 of August 1927—Jaca

I dream that I am waiting along with other people to take an examination for Legal Medicine. Maestre is on the board and he does not fail. I am anxious. In my mind I go over my facts and terrified I sense that I am very bad with toxicology and the laws of conscription, registrations.

I realize that I am 80 years old and it does not occur to me to note the strangeness of my position.

The distress awakens me.

Inconsistencies: Taking the examination being retired and not practicing medicine.

Noticing that there is a professor like Maestre almost a contemporary and kind and feeling primal terror.

Another dream: A lesson on the brain in a center for bullfighters and enthusiasts presided over by Romero Robledo. They believe that nerve centers are a kind of gelatin and that the soul is everything. I try to prove that the brain possesses a structure.

Dreadful inconsistency.

INCOMPREHENSIBLE DREAM

Jaca, 28 of July 1928

The women who accompany me are frightened seeing me surrounded by soldiers and I awaken lost. It was the first dream (approximately 3 in the morning).

No underlying nor provoking circumstances at all for this tragic fantasy. War had not been discussed; the walls themselves were a surprise to me.

Was reading the new Landrú (Pedro Rey) an influence? It is not likely. My readings before sleep were two chapters of The Nature of the Gods, by Cicero. I do not play the role of hero which is beyond me.

The entire dream was a creation, since I never pictured myself on such warlike adventures nor would they be likely given my peaceful nature.

DREAM

I do not know why my family, my brothers and sisters wished to enter blockaded Zaragoza.

I approached the walls and saw a rifle sticking out that I snatched in one motion from a sentry soldier half asleep.

He comes down machete in hand screaming and I take it out on him and shoot him dead. Having been discovered, panic spread throughout the base.

TWO DREAMS

29 of July 1928

I am on the Neckar river. Alhucemas. Wide raging current. Shores covered with forest partly cut back to form paths. Some snowy mountains in the distance that they tell me is the Neckar range. I go for a walk with someone else and I say to myself, I would gladly live here, in this magnificent wildnerness. But the cold awakens me.

Complete fantasy. I have not been in Alhucemas, and from familiar descriptions I knew that it is an unnavigable brook that irrigates some orchards. The mountain range, unusual. Besides I have not been there, I know almost nothing. Distortion, then, of images that I read, with fantastical and hyperbolic additions.

It is summer. I have not read geographical tales.

ANOTHER THAT IS REMINISCENT

I arrive in Madrid with my family and we look for a house on Montera street. Not finding one, some of us go ahead and find accomodations. The rest of us stay behind, not knowing where my wife and one of our sons are lodged. Anxiety and distress. We search for the ones who went ahead but do not find them. We hope to see them passing seated at the table of a café. Nothing. We stay in another house.

There is here a very distorted reminiscence of an incident that took place in Amsterdam 20 years ago.

DREAM

November 1928

I am preparing to get out of bed when Pittaluga comes to see me. He presents me with a book: a kind of dictionary of terms used in Pathology. I leaf through it quickly. I get up. He talks about investing funds. The usual considerations about the fall of the peseta and the need to buy houses in good condition and with commercial value. The interest on State money will be worth less every day. Pittaluga agrees.

Underlying causes: the well-known incident.

Current evocative causes: conversations had with my sisters whose heirs advised them against my advice to sell two houses, conversations from this summer recalled by my wife.

—No repressed desire. I neither buy nor sell buildings. Nothing unconscious at all.

[On the back of the page is written]:

The journals that are not continued are forgotten. In Germany and France there are many that died, when the driving force dies. Like life, it is necessary that it lives. 3 generations is a living thing. Like a mirror the entire contemporary medical movement has been reflected in its pages. In it the doctor has found information, salvational remedies and advice for his doubts and his worries.

DREAM

Argument about Jesus. I defend that he was a prophet, but a man, in front of people or another opinion.

Genesis, reading of [-----] where the [-----] and the Christian dogmas are refuted. A month before . . .

DREAM (ABOUT QUOTIDIAN THINGS)

November of 1928

I lecture on stereoscopic photography and I emphasize the well-known fact that the right proof should be placed on the left and other things all consistent but all common knowledge and familiar.

Underlying cause. The long orthographic habit, interrupted by old age and weariness.

Evocative cause. Having shown two or three visitors, one of them a photographer, stereoscopic photographs.

DREAM

I debate the ancient population of Spain against who knows who. I point out the 40 million of Marias Picarza.

I give 6 or 7 +++ melons [-----] of the Catholic Kings.

ANOTHER DREAM

23 of November 1928

I am seated on a pier on the shore. In the sea several children play with a boat full of stones. They are placed on top, the boat is drowned, a child disappears; two sailors who were next to [-----] look for him, but the child does not appear. I awaken.

Work of the imagination that I cannot attribute to anything except the adhesion of partial memories, joined with ingenuity. I find no underlying causes. My last reading was Athens (La Gréce) Band-Bovy. L'image de la Grece et de la Serbia. Photographic shadings. Paris. Fabre Souvenirs entomologique. Les epeires.

DREAMS

10 of December 1928

I give a talk with great spirit and energy in who knows what foreign university, and I say that histologists and physiologists must be weighed and not counted. That there are three classes of them, those who worship truth and having great experience know when to change opinion. There are not more than 10 or 12 of these; those who wish to be famous in order to succeed, but without seriousness and love of truth; and 3rd the iconoclasts, who deny or distort the facts by means of interpreting them, and whose ideal would be the [-----] of science and of all its prestige to be left alone with their machines, opinions and discoveries.

DREAMS (IN SIGÜENZA)

I am an auxiliary professor. Suddenly I receive direct orders from the dean to devote the last few minutes to osteology. Anxiety, distress ✳✳✳ upon reviewing the bones in my memory. I list those of the hand: scaphoids, capitate, and I did not know any more. Meanwhile the class is waiting for me, the students yell. I ask myself how I will teach bones if I have nearly forgotten them? Increasing distress and I awaken with a sense of wellbeing upon seeing that I am not a professor, I am old and no one is in charge of me.

Inconsistencies:

1. Imperiously demanding a 77-year-old retiree teach osteology.
2. Neither poor health nor lack of time to prepare myself occurring to me as possible excuses.
3. Forgetting of things that I knew; when I awaken, I recite the carpal and tarsal bones from memory with no mistakes.

(Obstruction of mnemonic centers).

Precedents: For 50 years I was an auxiliary professor and taught anatomy and other courses, according to the orders of the Dean (Zaragoza) and later chair of Anatomy in Valencia. But I received the teaching assignment a day in advance which allowed me to prepare myself.

Strange that I who learned all the details of osteology from my father from the ages of 12 to 15, would find myself hindered in things that I still know. It is, then, an inaccurate and fragmentary evocation of remnants of facts with distortions of those same facts, since if I had been asked to lecture on bones when I was an auxiliary, it would have been done passably and without preparation.

Where is the repressed desire? I do not see it. The desire was fulfilled 50 years ago and now I have other preoccupations. The dream, then, is a fragmented and misshapen evocation of some painful scene in my life as an auxiliary when I had to teach lessons in surgical or medical Pathology with little preparation, not in Anatomy which I knew well.

DREAM IN ACCORDANCE WITH FREUD

I dream that I am in the laboratory examining magnificent preparations of the reptile brain with the modified Golgi. I show them to the assistants. I show them some reptiles so that they might work on them. Then I pass through Belgium and I find myself with Meterlinck and fall into conversation about what he earns as a professor. He tells me that he does not know nor does it interest me. Good sign: that proves that you have income from other sources. I talk about Frederick and he says that he does not know him.

Inconsistencies: I do not know Meterlinck, and I believe that he is not a professor but rather a writer.

Cause. Could it be reading his books about bees, termites and last the Great [-----]? But how to explain that upon speaking with him I did not remember that he is a writer, knowing as I do many of his books and conferring upon him a professorship that he does not hold? This is an incoherent dream, not subject to the law of repressed desire, since I desire neither to travel nor to meet Meterlinck.

FANTASY

26 May 1929

Before the veronal and before 3:30.

Goes fast. Does it happen in the great hall of a theater?

I enter a hall where apparently there was a war between liberals and reactionaries. Before entering in a kind of foyer I come across several wounded men among others who display a bullet wound on the forehead and Lafora walks around saying, I have a serious injury. He wears no bandages. Unarmed I enter the great hall where shots are heard. Some enemies see me, but they do not shoot from the side where I am. Someone from the other side says: leave, so that nothing happens to you. Very arrogantly, I answer, shoot all you like, that they will take at most a few months off of my life. But they do not shoot. They say that it is not worth the trouble. In view of this I leave. The excitement awakens me.

It seemed like target practice rather than a battlefield. Nothing was compelling me to enter. And it seemed that the fight was of a political nature and was sustained between liberals and reactionaries.

Completely absurd. I did not see dead people.

Causes: The death of Enrique de Mesa from an embolism read earlier in the day. The execution by firing squad of a student who attempted to kill Valdemoros (Finland?). I do not understand it. I do not talk with anyone. My activities during the day have been peaceful; gone in an automobile to my orchard to pick sour cherries.

Inexplicable. I fell asleep reading a book [-----] by Julio Camba. I do suspect any repressed desire.

DREAM

29 of May 1929

We are in a theater or assembly hall. Meeting of the League of Nations. I attend with Cabrera unregistered. When we leave we leave with Gimeno who had made a beautiful speech. But I leave without an overcoat on. I have left my overcoat and I go in to look for it. I do not find it, but I find my cloak. We are alone away from the crowd, the three of us.

They tell me I wore an overcoat and not a cloak. Nevertheless the cloak was mine. I look for the overcoat again to no avail. I awaken.

Inconsistency: I do not attend theaters nor meetings and it would be wrong to wear a cloak and no overcoat. Both were left in the house.

Causes: papers with League of Nations speeches. Having read Amalio's speech. It is a real event, but I was not there. I do not even know if Cabrera attended.

I do not hit upon the interpretation. It was 3:03 in the morning before the veronal.

Readings Quevedo, The Great Tacaño, and Freud's theory of dreams.

A DREAM

16th day of August 1929
Temperature 80 degrees

I am in Valladolid and I enter the Faculty of Medicine. In a seminar room I write an application for the chair of Physiology despite being retired. The request is addressed to the Dean.

In case I am the lucky winner I visit one of the classrooms. My friend López García accompanies me, also retired and nonetheless practicing. And I find out that there are no benches. The students crowd together on foot. The building is new and beautiful.

Inconsistencies: There is no desire much less now that I am sick. [-----] of asking the dean for the chair and being a physiologist.

ANOTHER DREAM

I am in a social club, I drink coffee and while leaving I see that a cane has been exchanged for a kind of baton. I take hold of it and reach the automobile with ease.

Pure nonsense.

DREAM

13 of November 1929

I dream that I am writing a translated novel and struggling with the vocabulary. The translation is a little loose and I say to myself: "will I not I be critized?"

Precedents. I do not know, it has never occurred to me nor have I spoken about that with anyone.

ANOTHER

The same night

I fantasize that they put a strange electromagnetic apparatus on my head to make me sleep.

DREAM

December of 1929

There was a kind of pavillion where newspapers were sold and refreshments were drunk.

With sadness I see that the evening newspapers report the death of a writer much admired by me and a devoted friend. Agitation and difficulty falling asleep.

I read Cicero, then Quevedo, finally I fall asleep. I dream pleasant and indifferent scenes. Among other things that in a town next to Madrid we had rented a little house for the summer. The town has cottages, a market, and a shaded walk. Our house is comfortable and well situated. During the faltering and coherent dream I do not think about my friend. We are in winter. December. It is not the time for summer vacation.

It is curious that the next town over from Madrid does not look like ✻✻✻ Fuencarral nor Pozuelo, nor anyplace. It is a synthesis of fragments of several vacation towns. Without seeming like any of them. By its location to the north and it being flat it should be Fuencarral but it does not look like it.

I awaken at 9 after a bad night with severe insomnia.

Work of imagination on the town and house [-----].

Dora dreams that Padro has been shot. She does not give details.

Inconsistency. Padra is rich and happy and working. He was in his house two days ago.

There are no precedents. It does not have a premonitory character.

DREAM

18 of December 1929

I dream that I am competing in *oposiciones* for a chair and that I have an opponent. Locked in a department I draw the figures for the lecture on the blackboard. I go down to the seminar room with my opponent to give my talk when I think, but this is absurd. Why do I want to compete if I am a retired professor? And I awaken.

These are reminiscences of old *oposiciones* with variations on places, people. I do not remember what chair I competed for.

DREAM

23 of December 1929

I dream that I am making a catalogue of the books and magazines in the Laboratory completing it with the index of monographs.

The work is already done and it cannot be attributed to desire, at least now because unfortunately I do not read much, and we hire someone who does this work in order by author and subject.

[Written on the back]

Every generation that has not waged war desires war, in other words the governing and military classes. We must move the scales, we must sell ammunition and we must speculate with the soldier's hunger. As long as there are arms factories there will be war (see the United States).

Civil war as well stirred up by the jobless.

DREAM

I am in the Congress conference room, seated together with my wife and her two friends.

A self representative (not a delegate nor a senator from what I can recall) approaches and gives me a copy of the divorce law and another of the constitution. I read some articles from the one about divorce, but the delegate takes the copy away and he reads. Next I notice that there is a session and I peek in through one of the doors of the chamber while the delegate friend goes in to take his seat. The session begins . . . and I awaken.

Inconsistencies; Neither am I a delegate nor have I desired to be one.

My wife has been deceased for two years.

I am 79 years old.

Women are not allowed in Congress (meetings).

I am in Alicante.

Reading: Marmot and some of "In slippers, France Bronson.

Wishing for man not to be ungrateful, for friendship to persist, for love to endure and the [-----] is to want evolution and regression to stop, the two ✳✳✳ movements that [-----] men and worlds.

DREAM

I dream that in a boarding house in Madrid I run into an *oposiciones* candidate for lawyer. And in our conversation I say that I am going to compete in *oposiciones* for Anatomy in Zaragoza, to be close to my parents and siblings (—Well are You not already in Madrid? Yes, but I wish to leave the capital and change course).

Origin: Reminiscence of old *oposiciones* in Anatomy.

Inconsistencies: Being retired and aspiring to be a chair, without being able to be one. Wanting to go to Zaragoza, where I could have gone a long time ago and did not. Forgetting that I am 79 years old (or 75?); unsatisfied desire? It never was. To be a professor today? Neither, I feel weak, old and incapable of making a speech. What I desire is rest and solitude in order to read and write, my only two temptations.

DREAM

I look at a cathedral accompanied by who knows who and I see the stones covered (in ancient engraving) with the Fleurs de Mal by Baudelaire. It surprises me.

— Transmutation. I find myself at the table of a café and Azorín who is conducting who knows what survey, hands me a sheet of paper to write what I think about death and the hereafter. I excuse myself. My ideas, I reply, are not publishable. Let us work and let us stop with theologies, extremely smug. What is urgently necessary is that [-----] confidence by discretion and diligence and above all creating original science or industry, verses, novels, and paintings everyone makes; what only the greatest people do is contribute to the understanding of nature. This is the sole accomplishment that is respected. All the rest are purely entertainment.
— Cause: I had read the biography of Baudelaire.

DREAM

Taking advantage of some acquaintances' trip to the theater, we take over their house to develop some plates. There were two of us, one undoubtedly the son of the house. We take advantage of worn out trays, but nevertheless we resort to platters. There was no water in the improvised dark room and we used a jug from the dining room.

Our great trepidation not to stain the table of the dark room (some study) and to put the platters and jug in their place before the owners came back. 5 or 6 rather large plates were developed that had to wait for fixation due to lack of sufficient trays.

This is formed from reminiscent elements with creation from the imagination.

It is not desire, since for many years now I have a laboratory in my house and in the Institute, and the state of my health does not permit me to work nor do I have the desire to. My machines survive, but I do not use them, lacking desire.

On the other hand I remember more than once in my travels having developed in a boarding house, many years ago, but almost always alone.

Here the imagination works on elements of memories with a change of theme. Without any current or sentimental consideration. These were real many years ago. The scenes were very real and vivid.

DREAMS

In Bank of Spain and a friend came who was run (Astis?) approaches me and tells me that the Nuevo Mundo had published who knows what erroneous news about me. And then he joins up with his circle. Then I approach and say: I am not surprised because 8 days ago that same newspaper published the list of the senator elects for Madrid with portraits and Dr. D. José Rivera who died 4 years ago was included in it. This fact is accurate. One sees that memory is an exact reality copy in dreams. [-----] I saw the portrait of Reviera in the newspaper and not Rivera. The concrete fact is therefore faithfully recorded in the dream above all if it is a visual image of a person from a book or magazine.

DREAM

26 of May 1934

About histology.

I arrive at the laboratory after an absence of a few months. In my house I have applied the Ehrlich method to the brain and cerebellum (✳✳✳ [-----]). And after being fixed in Bethe's liquid I try in the abandoned laboratory to hydrate and set it in paraffin.

General commotion, the ingredients are missing, the ice for absolute alcohol, the xylol, the soft paraffin. With great surprise I notice that all the porcelain dishes and ✳✳✳ glass dishes are not only dirty but also coated with mold and even thickets of herbs (thyme, retama, [-----]). How is this possible, I shout. People are alarmed. I awaken.

Note. I have not used the Ehrlich method for more than 25 years. The laboratory [-----] by one of my students has good personnel and material.

Inconsistencies. No I had not asked for ice nor for paraffin and my complaint was useless. Absurd moreover that the porcelain dishes were covered in herbs.

[-----]

The contradiction is explained ✳✳✳ by the hypothesis of fallow cells.

FANTASY

I dream that I have hidden a check from my Bank checking account in a pile of sand on the outskirts of Madrid and that from a nearby mound I am surprised as in front of a number of curious onlookers a woman digs to find it and take it with her. Since I found myself on high ground nearby and I could not get down to stop it ✳✳✳ in the act without taking a dangerous leap and I shout at the woman. And from the excitement I awaken.

Underlying cause: the reminiscence of having hidden as a child some toy, drawing, or precious object between rocks in a field.

Determining: It does not exist.

Absurdity: Enormous. The illogic of hiding money in a pile of sand while having a checking account in the Bank or being able to keep it at home. It is a clear inconsistency.

DREAM

They call me from Paz's house in Madrid. I get there in two days. I forget, I ask a doctor who was living in the same house. And he tells me he has just died. He wanted You his friend to do an analysis of bile vomit. I do not perform tests, I respond. I feel deeply ashamed.

Real incident, it was years since Paz had died of cancer in Ávila. His survival and the change of illness were inconsistent.

Underlying incident: Spoke to a friend the previous day about the hepatic diseases cured in Vichy and Cestona from bold diagnoses.

Freud? Nothing.

DREAM IN JACA ON A FEVERISH NIGHT

I am in a Cathedral with Gómez Basquero. And seeing the religious ceremony I make comments about the vissisitudes through which Christianity has passed. To the surprise of my interlocutor I say that the religion of Yahweh has passed through various incarnations. First, the fierce and jealous cult of the God of Israel; then the doctrine of Jesus, next the [-----] of San Pablo and San Juan. Later on the work of the councils of Rome and finally the religion of the Jesuits. The spirit of Jesus is absent and I see nothing but pharisees and merchants of the temple. If Jesus were resurrected and lucky enough not to be locked up in a mental hospital with what righeous anger would he scorn his descendents.

I awaken.

The same night I am in ✳✳✳ London who knows for what. In the street I meet Decref and Pepe Botella who do not speak a word to me, I go into a boarding house where I suppose that ✳✳✳ I have been staying for days and I notice that behind the front door instead of stairs there is a rock one must climb. I ask the doorman the reason for that rock that one must crawl up to reach the first landing and his answer is to make the guests do gymnastics. This is the epitome of the inconsistency, for having been in London many times I have never seen anything like this.

That same night I had a dream about Azorín, who had presented an essay about El Cid to a certain dignitary. I went to get that dignitary to bring him to my house where his wife was waiting for him.

Inconsistencies and uninterpretable nonsense.

Let me note that I spent tonight reading until 3 in the morning about the Marseillan Landrú and his deeds, a graph of Madrid, the battle of the Invincible (the Globe). Nothing related to these readings was reproduced in the dream.

DREAM

Facile polemical lectures on philosophical science that last for hours and I have to awaken in order to avoid intense mental fatigue and to change the subject.

Capacity for expression. My wife awakens me by turning on the light.

DREAMING

A classification of sensory bases has been made. At first glance this classification is correct. The communicative and perceptive sensory fields are separated in different cerebral organs. But two or three categories of impressions almost always participate in the act of dreaming, the visual, the acoustic, and the tactile, not counting emotional phenomena. So for example a visual hallucination almost always exists in the dream as this entails a human scenario, acoustic and tactile hallucinations arise. We hear voices, we see people and landscapes, we are aware of our movements (kinesthetic feeling). And as a result [-----] except symmetry and logic we prefer the following that arranges hallucinations in order of complexity.

In every dream there is a psychic agglutinative. We would gladly call it imagination; but this acts consciously and selectively while the psychic or hallucinatory agglutinative acts without our permission pasting and fusing the most disparate scenes.

Another phenomenon is the exchange or phantasmagoria of subjects, the transforming agent that also works without our assent, even if the images are conscious. It could be called kaleidoscopic action.

DREAM

He was in his village, and he saw a horrible storm with hailstones like fists that caused disasters. We are in November.

Unknown evocation, qualifying causes, unknown.

DREAM

I attend an international Congress of International Law in Madrid. The President says that first we have to address what is dividing the legislations. A son of Flores de Lemus speaks on the matter. I take notes, there are 20 or 30 of us around the table.

Absurd. I have no desire to attend congresses nor do I understand a thing about this subject nor have I ever believed in the efficacy of these congresses. In international politics the strongest opinion is the only opinion.

Explanation, the recent Hague congress' suggestion of reparations?

DREAM

Oposiciones tribunal in Histology. It is Bertual, Tello, Cagigal [-----] in San Carlos and we choose the questions. I do not agree with the other candidates. On some topics I do.

Pure reminiscence.

DREAM

I cannot sleep, I leave the boarding house in an unfamiliar city in search of a pharmacy. I am looking for a product that is not veronal and whose name I do not know. What I take to be a pharmacy turns out to be a bakery.

More anxious I search along unfamiliar streets. And in a state of fatigue I awaken.

DREAM

I go with someone from my family to some small city and I buy land developments for not a lot of money. We talk about drawing up streets, selling plots.

I do not know to whom I speak and about what area. The blueprint for it does not resemble anything.

Occasion; having spoken days before with one of my sons-in-law about the business of land development and lamenting not having bought other lots next to my house when they were going cheap because of fear of spending and scarcity of resources.

DREAM

And late in the morning I dream that, when everyone from the staff of the Laboratory is gone, I was squatting down getting ready to count the money in a small cash box. Without my knowledge it becomes apparent that a thief is threatening me with a black object that I believed was a revolver. I awaken. I was not armed.

Inconsistencies: There is no cash box in the Laboratory nor is the money kept in a low drawer. I do not know how the thief infiltrated my room. I do not know the thief. I did not read about robberies in the newspaper. My readings before sleep were Cicero's [-----] about dreams and Quevedo, El Buscón, until I fell asleep. I do not see the fulfillment of a repressed desire.

GRANDDAUGHTER

House of wild animals. Many wild animals were eating her. I am not alive.

—

The bull had to go through a field and as he passed he gored your head and he bit into it and later it turned out that he had buried the head underneath the pillow.

—

A girl playing and they gave her a shove and an embankment she fell. It startled her awake.

—

She broke the head of a very pretty doll and replaces it with the head of a ragdoll that she painted eyes and the mouth. It was very ugly, but she liked it more.

—

Thieves come in. And I was saying to them: do not kill me, and they took out a revolver and then it turned out it was a toy to scare me.

—

In school the desks became beds and you were sleeping there. Visitors were coming and they were feeding you. The teacher brought you chocolate.

—

Cannibals. You were walking around an island and some black cannibals jumped out and they put you on the grill and poured oil. You, so peaceful. They were eating you and they were commenting and saying that the meat was hard and needed to fatten up still.

—

A cinema in the church. And by a ray of light through the roof I could see skulls and skeletons. She does not know any more. The cinema was the priest's doing.

TERESA

Escoriarza, La Libertad, 25th of May. The voice of wisdom has condemned the discoveries of Columbus, Gallileo, and Servet. No, Columbus is not considered to be a discoverer, but rather a bad governor. Neither is Gallileo for his discoveries, but rather because he insisted that the earth revolves around the sun, not his discovery but rather Copernicus' nor Servet for the circulation of blood but rather for denying the Trinity. For him there will only be one God. And Asuero is not disputed because he cures, but rather because he cures by suggestion, without admitting it and using a discredited and [-----] procedure of Pierre Bonnier.

DREAMS
Dora

2 in one night

That she was going through the street naked and the women were amazed at her robustness and beauty. She was not ashamed. Then she covered half of her body with a blanket and awoke.

Another dream: She was struck by an automobile and a horseman carried her in his arms to the free clinic. She was poorly covered, he got underneath her skirt, she was ashamed and was awoken by the nightmare.

Gracián

Criticón seeing everything for the first time (16 bk. I)

29. Curb of sand for the sea (what poet said it besides Gracían? Was it Quintana? I do not remember).

Strike but listen, said the philosopher to a tyrant of antiquity. Representative Estaucelin said it (Le radical 30th of October 1885)

To protect the swine is to protect us from ourselves. L'independence Belgue. 28 janvier 1910. It refers to a Belgian orator.

DREAM

I assist a pregnant woman and it goes well.

Some time later I find the couple and a child on Alcalá street; they greet me affectionately and I congratulate them on the child's good health.

Inconsistency: I have not practiced medicine, let alone obstetrics, for 40 years.

It has to do then with some memory of when I was attending, helping my father, some birth in Zaragoza or in Valencia.

PHOTOGRAPHIC DREAM

Dream: That Lipman briefed me on a kind of exposure, his invention for seeing relief, it was a photograph that one sees through a tube, one sees relief. Moving the apparatus in a certain way, multiple images could be seen.

It is strange that the house of this expert was not Lipman's house, it seemed more like Edisson's and he was clean-shaven.

On the floor I picked up two photographs that I believed [-----] but they did not have lenses.

All in all: many inconsistencies. There was a large audience.

— Other dreams: I sleep on the train and I hear noise and I am convinced that there is an earthquake and that the house is sliding into the abyss.
— I dream that I see figures and it occurrs to me to cover my eye and leave my hand there. I awaken and see the eye was covered. I had dreamed that I was doing the experiment without actually doing it.

TERRIBLE DREAM—TACTILE DREAM
(EVENING ESPRONCEDA)

I dream that they remove my skull and only skin covers the brain. I feel the contact of brain with skin and the falling of weight to one side, I hold it back with my hands awaiting the doctor who will make a protective skullcap for me out of who knows what. I find it very natural that they have removed the skull and I remember another dream about the same thing in which my skull grew back again and the cavity was reinforced. I cannot understand the operation, and I find it very natural for it to be done and for the brain to be covered with skin without further precautions. I go for a walk around the room and am alarmed and I awaken when I see that my brain is falling out. (The scene happens in the house on the street where the Zaragoza Hospital is). My wife ✳✳✳ is alarmed.

(I have dreamed this other times). It is surprising to walk and not fall, unconscious. My hands placed on my head touch something smooth that is moving. I alert my wife who does not know what to put on me; I am missing my discarded skull. It is an operation that I deem natural and common. Distress at last and I awaken. As soon as I want to try and touch, I am not able to because I am awake.

Precursor, having seen the brain in an autopsy? I do not believe that having seen a trepanation years ago (was it on the skull of Espronceda? Retina theory impossible here.

They are emotional dreams, they do not lend themselves to explanation. They awaken me immediately.

DREAM

I was in Tangiers and I was visiting the son of a Jew who had dislocated an arm. The house and the race were Jewish. The last dream was the second visit, and the strange thing is that the first was in the previous dream, and that upon talking with the head of the family I ✦✦✦ hardly remembered what I was going to do there; and he reminded me of the previous visit, saying that the son was well.

DREAM

Waiting in Pitaluga's house.

The sitting rooms and patio garden full of aristocratic people. I leave with my pants falling down and embarrassed.

Sea expedition at 4 in the morning. Near the port I fall into the water with a child. I drown and I awaken.

Now dreaming I have seen clear relief walking down the stairs, in other words, stairs depth as well as natural colors. Everything was very bright and rich in detail. There were new things that did not seem to be copies of sensations, but rather new sensations or a combination of basic sensations.

FANTASY WITH AUTO-OBSERVATION

I come to a store that is at the back of a large entrance hall; it was Galvi's. I thought that it would be color photographs only; it was meant to be innovative; I go up some stairs to the mezzanine; I see an entrance display window to the right an enormous picture, in color a color photograph of more than a meter [-----] Lumiere which progressively loses color and turns into a relief sculpture, gray tones like those of painted plaster flowers.

When I go into the store I trip and break a glass and the people inside scream. I go in to pay for it (this has never happened) and the store previously filled with photographic things I find converted into a boutique. For the most part the floor is filled with models for women's panties. It is difficult to move. There are mannequins. I see a group of ladies and I confront the one who seems to be the owner. She has brown hair and a large nose, healthy almost red complexion. She wears a dark suit, almost greenish; she is less than a meter from me; I see as far as [-----]. In that moment I say to myself: Here we have a good opportunity to determine two things: the color, the relief and the [-----] disappears and changes the image precisely as

Delage and Berngson say. Good relief but the image changes; the woman ages and wrinkles, the hands are deformed and blurred, the mouth ✱✱✱ turns into a snout, the mass of flesh seems to transform into the palette of a painter or better yet into a gray out of focus face with no details. The clothes lose their creases, are unevenly wrinkled, take on a gray black tone, loses light and finally everything is degraded before fading into black and I awaken.

This is notable; because I did not see the image resolve itself into luminous points in [-----] phenomena; for witnessing the deformation and the degradation of the image, for corroborating relief once again. In short because of the synthetic action of the image. There were no familiar people, perhaps there were elements of people but there was no single person; there is creation with primitive sensory elements.

DREAM

I am in Cadiz, and in a house overlooking the sea. I believe the widow of an old friend, Martín Virgil (?) lives there.

I go out to the wall and throw myself into the water in order to reach land. But the depth is great and I run the risk of drowning. I ask where the sea is not as deep and they point at another angle. Another dip and once again I recede. With the distress of not being able to get to the Penninsula I awaken.

Inconsistencies:

1. I have forgotten that Cadiz is not an island, but a peninsula and that one can reach the land by railroad.
   I have forgotten that the sea in the bay of Cádiz is very deep.
   I have forgotten that there are motor boats to go to San Lúcar, to the port.

Causes: Impossible, it has been more than 57 years since I have seen the city and I cannot explain having dreamed that I was there.

Neither do I see the utility.

It is an imaginative creation with fragments of memories and pertaining to different time periods.

EROS DREAM

3 a staircase—Hand—People go down, we run away. Somebody falls; hurts nose. Cross country in search of the others. Only two [-----]. Shocks. They were friends. A [-----].

Circumstances: extremely late reading and conversation. Disturbed mind. Nightmare that awakens me. 3 a.m. All implausible.

SCIENTIFIC DREAM

Two students, one female +—+ arriving abroad are trying to prove to me that in normal blood plasma there live millions of almost ultramicroscopic organisms to whom we owe the nutritive properties of the blood. They tell me having cultivated them in vitro and showing them to me. I object.

Reminiscences of views on the parasitism of organisms read a long time ago. Like lichens the organism would be a mix of mushrooms and seaweed.

Determining? No. It is a deformed memory.

ARCHAEOLOGICAL DREAM

My wife and I are in ancient Rome. It is dark. We leave the inn by car to see the city. After driving a while we lose track of the inn. We cannot find the way back. My wife goes ahead. I do not know how to find her. How I long for a boarding house! The distress causes me to awaken.

Causes, I read Lucretius. Reminiscence of a journey to Holland during which a baggage check caused me lose my wife, who along with a few delegates was a few hours ahead of me.

Simulations that came from these things, pg. 179 in order to explain vision.

I am not thinking about modern Rome, but rather the ancient city.

Freud? Nothing.

Memory of Martial? Perhaps. All creation.

EXPERIMENT WITH OPTICAL DREAMING

[Drawing]

An object that is covered with small discal or linear screens should not be seen in a movement of well-timed convergence. And vice versa the whole object should be seen.

Marked with holes across the screen following the visual lines of convergence.

DREAM OF DORA

Dreams by Autosuggestion

People that consult the code of dreams sometimes dream in accordance with the responses of that code.

A woman dreams about dolls or about children and finds in the code that she should renounce her marriage. In others that she goes down the stairs. The interpretation is that she will go from bad to worse and that there will be no end to her misery. These dreams coinciding with the responses from the code should be attributed to suggestion, and they are among the few that validate Freud, since she who dreams with dolls usually longs for a good marriage. The code is nonsense.

But these dreams, consistent with desire are very rare, even in those young people in whom the libido is very imperious.

DREAM

I rent a consultation room in the same apartment building as Marañon. I sleep alone there. The following morning Marañon calls and tells me: living together does not matter, when I have a patient who is doubtful or suspicious of not being well I will send him to you.

In the morning, an unfamiliar woman who turns out to be the wife of an auxiliary employee from [-----] makes me breakfast and tells me that it was wrong of us to assign her husband to Valladolid.

Dreadful inconsistencies. Cause: an article that I read from the book intersexual States. All the rest is inexplicable.

Because I neither visit, nor intend to visit, nor dedicate myself to [-----] studies, nor was I going to stay in the borrowed house of a friend for a visit. It is, therefore ✳✳✳ inconsistent. As for desire, null and void. At my age my only desire is to have a bit of health. Readings: The tragic sentiment of life, by Unamuno and the natural History (?) of man, by Virey. 1353 (?) edition, where incidentally I find he brings up the problem of eugenics and the union of a monkey with a woman to create a new race.

Arrival at [-----]. Customs visit. Scene of exchange with a shopkeeper from whom I buy a guide to the city. I pay with francs.

— Dissocation from the family. They go ahead of me in a car or boat where [-----] and I remain alone, not knowing where to look for my siblings.

(Real incident: the one from Holland).

DREAM

23rd of October

They present me with an enormous book about Histology with a colossal wealth of color figures. I skim through it and I see that it is impossible to bring it to the seminar room and show it to the students. It comes from Valencia from a certain Peset, the chair of general pathology. Magnification of something *＊＊* seen, but adding work of the imagination.

I search for dwarves to study them and they provide me a collection of dwarf women, atrophic, none of whom reach 50 centimeters. I want to buy them, almost all of them speak with a high-pitched and almost imperceptible voice. I wish to carry them with me and then the dream vanishes.

Pure imagination. They did not look like real dwarves.

No desire; I have never had the tendency to study the psychology of freaks.

DREAM—SIESTA

I dream that I am sitting around the table after dinner among friends. Astronomy comes up and I go on about the planets. I speak about astral collisions. A black star, perhaps a planet, collides with another. It starts to boil. It vaporizes. Goodbye civilization, science, culture, religion. Nothing is more tragic.

Incidental. In the morning I learned that a bus near [-----] was destroyed leaving its 24 occupants who were happily coming from France injured. The surgeon amputated arms, sewed flesh.

DREAM

I dream that I debate the course of the (?) bundles of the bulb with a Frenchman. I justify my preference for rat, in some cases cat and rabbit. He shows me sympathetic nervous system preparations in lengthways sections from rats and other animals.

—Causes: None. In the summer I do not talk about that with anyone. It could only have been an allusion made by Benteus about optic pathways the previous day in a lecture alluding to my work; but I did not hear it and I addressed neither the optic pathways nor the retina with the Frenchman in his laboratory.

DREAM

It is summer. I sleep in my own villa. Large window to the countryside. A (?) hand appears and strips the linens from the bed. I shout: Thieves! I awaken.

So I dream that I am sleeping and they rob me.

DREAM ABOUT WRITING

Another. A friend cites a paragraph from a [-----] of mine that he is transcribing. He gives me the manuscript in case I wish to correct or add something. I take it; I cross out [-----] words, phrases; I dedicate myself [-----].

But I am not satisfied. I slave away to improve the style. With this distress I awaken.

ABSURD DREAM

To the American professor, to whom I had shown microbes using standard methods, I show preparations of the semicircular pathways in birds (the adult pigeon) which under the microscope revealed some giant multipolar nerve cells with straight branches. Bones were showing up in them that were similar to those of Halmgren.

It has been a long time since I have worked on microbes and as for these multipolar cells they are pure fantasy. It did not even occur to me to think that the (?) vestibular cells are in Scarpa's ganglion and are bipolar. There is, then, amnesia of facts commonly known, fantasmal creation of others.

The American was in Madrid. It has been a month since I touched a microscope.

ANOTHER

That I am in Paris studying botany, observing the synthesis of plant and embryos, making sections in the house of a botany professor whose street I could not remember: that I walk around lost, searching for it.

—Elements of hallucination. I was in Paris with [-----], but studying nervous diseases.

Inconsistencies: I have never studied botany and I would have liked to learn it. This is one thing Freud is right about.

Note that what was read immediately before is never dreamed: [-----] of Lafora, Initiation into philosophy by Faguet, Philosophy of Laertius, news from Journals and newspapers. Never what is most recent, what has immediate and precise memories.

DREAM

I dream that I am bored and go to America on a shoddy Spanish boat. (?) Sanchez Moguel accompanies me. Clouds accumulated on the horizon resemble an imaginary city. The boat's movement. I get seasick. Sanchez recites hendecasyllabic verses to me. A rocky and red coast appears, no green. They tell me, it is the start of the Canaries. At the sight of the land and the picturesque scenery I awaken.

1. I do not wish to go to America to which I have been invited and I fear the tropical climate.
2. Underlying causes: a trip that I read about by Brousson to Buenos Aires in which he tears Anatole France to pieces.
3. Deformed objective amnesiac elements. My two previous journeys to America, one at 22-years-old and the other at 49.
4. Censorship: null and void, I have no desire at all to go.

DREAM

That I go out to the provinces with other professors for a pedagogical tour. I talk about secondary education in who knows what center after other speakers. I point out its defects and its tendency to explore those vocations that advance the synthesis of general culture.

Why? The reason is that recently I had read a book on The History of Pedagogy [-----]. In any case it is a question that I have touched on only *** of the past in one of my books (Advice . . .) and in some way was the current object of my thoughts.

Two events from the day were: that a nephew won an appointment; that I had to fire a Chauffer for failure to fulfill his duty; that I spoke in the Laboratory about errors relating to the Golgi apparatus and the lack of foreign attention to this.

DREAM

I am coming from France, I am delayed for minutes in the last station and when I board the train to Spain ✳✳✳ I find the door closed on a cliff. I beg a Frenchman to let me pass; he says that the train is just about to leave; that I will not get there; I go in; I leap onto a moving minerals car, they want me to throw me off, but the train is already running and I continue into Spain.

Where, I do not recognize the international line, platform and gate. Is it Canfranc?

Inconsistencies. I no longer travel. I do not understand my hurry. I only remember my ✳✳✳ mania for traveling in [-----] and lingering in stations sometimes missing the train.

Freud? None of that.

DREAM

I dream that I am searching for a rare specimen, a tumor with radiated cells similar to [-----] and once found I make sure to place it in a special compartment of a cabinet careful not to lose it among thousands of preparations. There are a number of people advising me to take special care.

DREAM

I do *opisiciones* [-----] Anatomy chair and I am twenty-four years old [-----] inconsistencies, absolutely useless, it is explained by memories.

DREAM

I am invited to the house of an engineer. His wife watches me eating heartily. She is surprised and she congratulates me because she had heard rumors that I was sick on a diet and I was eating very little. We were talking about her husband, a man from the staff at the school whom I did not know. Roll call of unknown faculty and sincerely I say: forgive me, I do not know the professors from the civil engineering school very well.

Inconsistencies: It has been years since I have eaten outside the house. I am not familiar with any engineer's wife intimately enough that they would invite me to eat.

—But one would say, You are sick You usually have no appetite. Since You are well, thus your dream is the fulfillment of desire.

But in my dream there is no element of [-----] that can be interpreted by Freud. And the others, the distressing ones? Shall we resort to unconscious memories? But this destroys Freud's hypothesis. Whether or not distressing scenes from the past come to consciousness, there is no fulfillment of any desire here. And one must be very keen and very specious (?) in order to see a desire realized in 80 out of 100 of my dreams.

Other times I teach a lesson or give a lecture.

Desire? None. It is work and in my situation more. Is it that I desire to fulfill it? No.

But even if it were true it would explain my hypothesis better. It is an acquired habit that has not been carried out for 5 years. The cerebral cells affected by this task are resting, they have an excess of sensory, motor, and ideational memories and they are relieved of their overstimulation. Let us note the perfect logic of the lectures.

HYPNAGOGIC HALLUCINATIONS

Maury says that hypnagogic hallucinations almost always deal with figures smaller than natural miniatures. The eye discerns the falsehood. Sometimes they are vibrant and they have more relief than in reality. He never has seen images of a normal size (I have: In hypnotism they are always of a normal size). The images are *-*-* [-----] but in a waking state they do not have a hallucinatory character and in dreams they do.

DREAM

30th of July

In a discussion with a friend from the Faculty of Sciences I talk about the flaws of the auxiliary faculty, about the capricious accumulation of appointments, about people without a vocation, *-*-* lifelong auxiliaries who are stiff and old, without aspirations or illusions.

Underlying causes: None. It is explained by ostracism from the faculty.

DREAM

I read visitor Ants, an illustrated book.

And I dream that I see ants that visit anthills in the walls and kill their sisters from another species, leaving. But sometimes they cannot and they stay between the slabs of a wall with part of the bounty.

—Some feverishness.

I take veronal afterwards, it is 3:30 in the morning.

DREAM

We are in Mexico. They invite me to paint the president of the republic's wife? and her sister. Both pure Indians. One of them is expecting. Her breasts prominent, her arms fleshy, her tanned face indicating the race and her pregnancy. Before finishing the portrait the Saxon nurse arrives, like the British or Americans? The outfit of the president's daughter is scantily clad, half savage.

I awaken.

Causes. Reading an article the previous day about Mexico where hatred of Spain is demonstrated in response to a proposal for a statue of Isabel the Catholic. It talks about the fact that it is going to be proposed to Parliament any day.

Is it my revenge? But I am not a painter nor have I been in Mexico nor do I feel animosity towards the President. Sympathy rather. It is about nothing more than an oil portrait in indigenous clothes.

I do not understand it. There must be influence from recent readings, in this case.

Freud. In the dream we experience surprise upon discovering the child who [-----] with its impulses.

In the dream there are preferences for what is recent and what is neutral and in Freud there are infantile memories we do not have at our disposal in the waking state.

DREAM

Silvia. That she married a priest and a friend at the same time in a town near Cercedilla. She does not know which.

—

Another, that she dreamed that Dora had married a drone (slacker) and that she went to his house and he taught her how honey is made.

—

Dora dreams that she marries a girlfriend, and that after arriving home they say: we are married now, have to work now to earn a living.

DREAM

I embark on a polar journey as an employee of ✳✳✳ some company or another. I cross France in order to search for a lost expedition. In who knows what country I take 1 with a ticket for 2, and with the anxiety of being discovered I awaken.

No preparations at all. No desires to travel, impossible because of illness. Lack of training in polar affairs. I have no idea where I am going or why I am going alone. All illogical.

Could it be that I sleep without a cap and this has given me a chill?

DREAM

I have written a treatise on modern physics that I am proud of and I hear from the press about the objections and corrections that everyone made.

Absurd: Never did I have such a crazy desire, even though I like physics.

Current project: a book of Histogenesis.

✳✳✳ Desired project and real desire: having time for the complete Works, and bringing to light my observations about dreams, the problem of immutability, my little philosophical jests.

[Written on the back]

DREAM

D. Antonio is killed and I am told to do his autopsy. And I do it in transversal slices, placing him in formol. He was undressed and I call the family to give them the 3 pesetas that he was carrying.

Inconsistency: ✳✳✳ died in Córdoba three years ago from vomiting blood.

That same night I toil at drawing water from a well with a pump placed in the hall instead of the elevator. Red water. I awaken.

DREAM

That Pérez de Ayala presents in the Church a play of his for fans among whom are two typists in my Laboratory to whom when asked I give relevant details about his family and orphanhood and achievements. That one of them is married and the bachelorette is on the verge of being married. I do not recall the details of the performance and the name of the comedy.

Inconsistencies. The church, Pérez de Ayala writing *** works for the theater and girls from a laboratory performing despite being completely unaware *** that they have such interests.

Repressed desire or metamorphosed symbolism, none. It is an ordinary game of the imagination. Of the people I remember above all Pérez de Ayala, admirable [-----].

All in all, a neutral dream, which says nothing and cannot be interpreted by Freud's hypothesis.

Dora dreams that she drives in an automobile with her mistress on a grass road and finds diamond earrings. She puts them on. It rains in torrents and they get to an inn to wait for the rain to stop. She cannot remember anything more (This favors Freud).

———

That I am in a café in a way station at night and surrounded by buildings and labyrinths to such an extent that it is impossible to see the direction of the departing train.

I confront the owner and tell him that he should put arrows indicating the exit to serve as a guide at night. He claims that he does not have the money. I give him 5 duros and he says that they will be painted on the façade. The train is from Zaragoza to Madrid and perhaps the station is [-----].

Reminiscence of being student in which I had to wait for the train and [-----] trains at night.

Here there is a desire but retrospective and altruistic since now I never stop in canteens on the track anymore.

DREAM

I go into Portugal (a city on high) and I search for a friend so that he can publish a book for me. I enter and leave for the border on foot, with no obstacles. I see the friend and I do not even greet him. I see Englishmen that I already met in Madrid. I think that everyone is making the return trip from Sevilla Madrid Portugal Sintra.

All inconsistencies.

Another dream: I discuss color photography.

MY NURSE

1. That she eats chocolate and believes it is a good omen.
2. That she mounts a horse and wins first prize in a race.

DREAM

I dream that I come to Turégano by autombile, I see the Castle.

Inconsistencies. I see the color of rocks, shops stuck to the wall. I have never been to Segovia.

Evocation. The previous day I drove by automobile to Pozuelo.

DREAM

That I read Isadora. And I had read it the days before. Spectacular, terrible book. Like the truth, a mix of sensuality, glory and death.

DREAM

I am in a boarding house where at night secretly I cut slices of medulla for Nissl staining. I keep the slices and the sections dried in my vest. ✳✳✳ I set them aside to stain in the laboratory. It does not occur to me to keep them in their alcohol bottles. I do not know how I came to have a microtome.

Foolish act. I go to a library (not mine) and secretlly tear out some pages of an uncompleted language dictionary, to make an alcoholic extract with them. The absurd act is witnessed by Dr. de Vicente, dead 25 years ago from cancer. It does not even occur to me to be surprised by the extraordinary apparition of my friend Vicente, which seems to me like a natural thing.

Precursors. During the day in the laboratory I fixed some cat tissues with different liquids, and in the afternoon (it was Sunday) I drove with my family by automobile to Pozuelo. None of this explains explains the dream (I awoke at 4 in the morning). The extinction of Dr. Vicente's image was the only thing I could not remember; it was a blurred image, not evoked for long, and I do not usually practice the Nissl method. Commemorative, resting, or neglected cells? It could be. In any case there is no explanatory theory and this one itself is not complete; since there are many millions of sensory images not evoked for a long time. Why this and not other memories? Why the nonsense about the dictionary earlier? A fabricated act? Why the coalescence of heterogenous memories unconnected to real life in the present?

At night I washed pieces set aside to be cut; but I do it frequently. Everything sharp and well-colored. Perfect relief.

DREAM

I am in bed. The doctor is preparing to perform a tracheotomy on me. I have difficulty breathing. I see the imposing instrument.

Precursor. It can only be an article by García Tapia that I read 20 days before about a girl on whom he had to perform the operation with a foreign body and whom suffocating he brought by automobile several times to Madrid.

DREAM

Return to childhood.
I venture across Madrid accompanied by a maid (the current one). On the street we run into a female acquaintance entering her house. I furtively snatch a cluster from her trained vine (on the door); she gets angry and I start running. I cross several streets, Fuencarral and Hortaleza, among others, and I get to my house located in the area around Arch of Saint Maria street and I hide there. Meanwhile, my maid accompanies the woman who was coming in the same direction, probably placating her and excusing me. I awaken.

Inconsistencies.

1. Anachronism, today's maid and mischief from the past.
2. I did not grow up in Madrid, the first time that I came I was 22-years-old.
3. Grapes are no longer my favorite dish, I almost never eat them.
4. Neither I nor my family has ever lived on Arch of St. Maria street.
5. In Madrid there is not a single grapevine on the central streets much less on the doors.

All pure nonsense with no purpose.

Game of imagination that has ✳✳✳ combined a scene taking elements from different times.

WELLS—DREAMS

1056

Dunne says that some dreams are anticipations of future events. Upon awakening he analyzes the dreams and records them.

He says that a considerable portion of our dreams appear to be based on experiences that took place in the immediate past; most are false interpretations of corporeal states (the cold of an exposed thigh evokes a bath of cold water) and others (psychoanalysts say they correspond to repressed complexes, Wells says). But Dunne adds that a considerable complex stays in [-----] that anticipates experiences of the immediate future.

Perhaps, Wells says they are coincidences; and there are dreams with anticipations that proved wrong.

Telepathy; thought transmission at a distance (wireless).

Murray and his daughter: One observer concentrates his attention on a book or painting in a separate room and the the other receives the transmission in another. Sir Olivier Lodge has done it with drawings; they are surprising coincidences, Wells says, difficult to explain without resorting to thought transmission.

For these cases Richet accepts a 6th sense without special organs.

Others explain it with hyperaesthesia.

Others with parallelism and coincidence.

Attuned minds that live close together follow similar pathways of mental association and respond with similar patterns of excitation (flights of social birds and movements of convivial herbavores, as Wells explains).

Wells says that professional magicians imitate it and that truthful stories have emphasis and exaggerations (almost all of us ✳✳✳ prefer to tell a story that accentuates characteristics to not having anything notable to say.

(The public only hears about telepathic triumphs that are achieved and not foiled).

Wells objects that with chess players, bridge players, or in sensitive communication, or in court, or in the bedroom, mental laxity is required for the message to arrive, while for all practical purposes the human skull is opaque.

Nevertheless he is not completely dimissive and with reservations he affirms that the sociability of bees, ants, collective social emotions of population X are capable having had [-----]. But the cult of personality goes against them.

One believes that they are creations of the unconscious (Wells).

GLOSSARY

Advice *Advice for a Young Investigator.*

Atheneum The Atheneum in Madrid is a historic center for literary, artistic, and scientific culture, home to a library, assembly hall, and plenty of space for *tertulias*, where prominent intellectuals such as Cajal attended.

Azorín The pseudonym of José Augusto Trinidad Martínez Ruiz (1873–1967), a prominent Spanish literary figure and friend of Cajal.

Berngson Misspelling of the name of Henri-Louis Bergson (1859–1941), an influential French philosopher who published articles on hypnosis, dreaming, and other metaphysical topics.

Blas Cabrera Blas Cabrera y Felipe (1878–1945) was an internationally recognized Spanish physicist whom Cajal had convinced to abandon law and start a career in science.

Criticón *El Criticón* is an allegorical Spanish novel by Balthasar Gracián from the middle of the seventeenth century. Gracián, an Aragonese Jesuit monk and philosopher, was a favorite writer of Cajal.

Delage Yves Delage (1852–1920) was a French biologist whom Freud cites in *The Interpretation of Dreams*. Delage believed that dreams are derived from regular sensory impressions, inhibited during the day but released during sleep. However, his associationalist model, in contrast to Freud, does not attribute psychic importance to these dynamics but, rather, explains the phenomenon by the activity of neurons.

Dora Dora Ballano was Cajal's last housekeeper.

Dunne John William Dunne (1875–1949) was a British aeronautical engineer and philosopher. In his book *An Experiment with Time*, he claimed to have precognitive dreams.

Ehrlich Paul Ehrlich (1854–1915) was a German scientist who invented a method to stain living cells, which Cajal borrowed. Ehrlich and Cajal were collegial friends for more than two decades, until the Great War separated them and Ehrlich died.

gangue A geological term meaning rock or mineral matter that appears in the same vein or deposit with metallic ore but is valueless.

Golgi Camilo Golgi (1843–1926) was an Italian scientist whose revolutionary histological technique, *la reazione nera* ("the black reaction"), Cajal utilized and improved in order to facilitate discoveries of the nervous system. Golgi was an invincible reticularist and therefore Cajal's rival; both were awarded the Nobel Prize in 1906 for their contributions to the field of neuroanatomy.

Gregorio Marañon Gregorio Marañon (1887–1960) was a former student of Cajal and a famous doctor and scientist who met Freud in person.

Isadora Isadora Duncan (1877–1927) was a legendary dancer, whose memoir *My Life* is likely the book to which Cajal is referring.

Maury Louis Ferdinand Alfred Maury (1817–1892), a forerunner to Freud whom Cajal admired and cites, systematically studied the effect of external stimuli on dreams by observing thousands of his own.

Jaca A small city in the Alto Aragón region of Spain where Cajal's father sent him as an adolescent to a religious boarding school for aspiring doctors.

Julio Camba Julio Camba (1886–1962) was a prominent Spanish journalist who was known at the time for traveling to other countries and reporting satirical observations of other cultures and his own.

La Esfera A weekly review of Spanish culture.

Lafora Gonzalo Rodríguez Lafora (1886–1971) was a neuropsychiatrist and pupil of Cajal with whom Germain, the transcriber of these dreams, worked closely.

Maestre Aureliano Maestre de San Juan (1828–1890) was one of the fathers of Spanish anatomy who taught Cajal, introduced him to histology, and preceded him as the Chair of Anatomy.

melons Most likely an error for *millónes, or millions.*

Oposiciones Competitive examinations that determine lifetime public service appointments. *Oposiciones* required a formal presentation and head-to-head debate, both of which were judged by a bureaucratic tribunal not immune to political and personal bias.

orthographic Most likely an error for *photographic.*

Pittaluga Gustavo Pittaluga Fattorini (1876–1956) was an Italian–Spanish pathologist whose work Cajal and his school admired and who met Freud personally.

pts. An abbreviation for *pesetas.*

Retina theory Cajal's findings on blind patients showed that the retina is not involved in visual dreaming—that as long as a person has visual memories, he or she can generate impressions.

Richet Charles Richet (1850–1935) was a French physiologist who not only won the Nobel Prize and made enduring contributions to mainstream science but also was influential throughout his career in promoting research in anamolistic psychology and parapsychology, allegedly having introduced hypnosis to Jean-Martin Charcot as an intern at the Salpêtrière.

Tagore The appearance of the great Indian poet Rabindranath Tagore (1861–1941) in a dream provokes Cajal to say that he "detests" poetry, but he fails to mention that when he was young he used to write verses, which are presented in the "Unedited Writings" volume of Durán Muñoz and Alfonso Burón's biography.

tertulia A ritual gathering for intellectual conversation and Cajal's vital means of social contact, which he called "the diastole to the systole of work." Cajal gave up this favorite activity after he was diagnosed with cerebral arteriosclerosis. He penned *Café Chats* as a record of memorable experiences after his favorite haunt, the Café Suizo, was demolished in 1920.

the theory of disuse An associationalist theory or law proposed by American psychologist Edward Thorndike (1874–1949) stating that the associations between cells that are more frequently active will be stronger and therefore more easily evoked, and vice versa.

"the well-known incident" The Great Depression.

veronal or **barbitol** The first commercially available barbiturate, for relief from "insomnia induced by nervous excitability."

you The second person pronoun *Usted*, a contraction of the Spanish title *your honor*, is used in formal address.

Wells Probably the science fiction author H. G. Wells (1866–1946).

BIBLIOGRAPHY

Alonso Buron, Francisco and Garcia Durán Muñoz. *Cajal: vida y obra*, 2nd edition. Barcelona: Editorial Científico-Médico, 1983.

Andres-Barquin, Pedro J. "Ramón y Cajal: A Century After the Publication of His Masterpiece."*Endeavour*25,no.1(2001),13–17.doi:10.1016/s01609327(00)01334-x.

Aviv, Rachel. "Hobson's Choice: Can Freud's Theory of Dreams Hold Up Against Modern Neuroscience?" *The Believer* (October 2007). http://www.believermag.com/issues/200710/?read=article_aviv.

Barbeito Varvela, Manuel. "Spanish and Spanish–American poetics and criticism." In *The Cambridge History of Literary Criticism: Volume IX, Twentieth-Century Historical, Philosophical and Psychological Perspectives*, edited by Crista Knellwolf and Christopher Norris. Cambridge, UK: Cambridge University Press, 2001.

Bentivoglio, Marina and Paolo Mazzarello. "The Anatomical Foundations of Clinical Neurology." Chapter 12 in *History of Neurology*, edited by Stanley Finger, François Boller, and Kennth L. Tyler, from *Handbook of Clinical Neurology*, vol. 95, edited by Michael J. Aminoff, François Boller, and Dick F. Swaab. Amsterdam: Elsevier, 2010.

Bogousslavsky, J. "Sigmund Freud's evolution from neurology to psychiatry: evidence from his La Salpêtrière library." *Neurology* 77, no. 14 (2011), 1391–1394. doi:10.1212/wnl.0b013e31823152a.

"Brain Initiative" (September 30, 2014). https://www.whitehouse.gov/share/brain-initiative.

Bush, George. "Decade of the Brain, 1990–1999, Proclamation 6158" (July 17, 1990).

Cajal's Degeneration and Regeneration of the Nervous System, translated by Raoul M. May. New York: Oxford University Press, 1991.

Calderón de la Barca, Pedro. *Life Is a Dream*, translated by Gregary Racz. New York: Penguin Classics, 2006.

Calvo Roy, Antonio. *Cajal: Triunfar a toda costa*. Madrid: Alianza Editorial, 2007.

Cannon, Dorothy F. *The Explorer of the Human Brain*. New York: Henry Schuman, 1949.

Cohen, David. *Freud on Coke*. London: Cutting Edge Press, 2012.

Colucci-D'Amato, L., V. Bonavita, and U. di Porzio. "The End of the Central Dogma of Neurobiology: Stem Cells and Neurogenesis in Adult CNS." *Neurological Sciences* 27, no. 4 (September 2006), 266–270.

De Carlos, Juan. *Ramón y Cajal: una familia aragonesa*. Zaragoza: Departamento de Cultura y Turismo, 2001.

De Carlos, Juan and María Pedraza, "Santiago Ramón y Cajal: The Cajal Institute and the Spanish Histological School." *Anatomical Record* 297 (August 14, 2014), 1785–1802. doi:10.1002/ar.23019.

De Cervantes Saavedra, Miguel. *Don Quixote*, translated by Edith Grossman. New York: Harper Perennial, 2005.

de Rijcke, Sarah. "Drawing into Abstraction: Practices of Observation and Visualization in the Work of Santiago Ramón y Cajal." *Interdisciplinary Science Reviews* 33, no. 4 (December 2008), 287–311. doi:10.11.79/174327908X392861.

DeFelipe, Javier. "Brain Plasticity and Mental Processes: Cajal Again." *Nature Reviews Neuroscience* 7, no. 10 (2007), 811–817. doi:10.1038/nrn2005.

DeFelipe, Javier. "Cajal and the Discovery of a New Artistic World: The Neuronal Forest." *Progress in Brain Research* 203 (2013), 201–220. doi:10.1016/B978-0-444-62730-8.00008-6.

DeFelipe, Javier. *Cajal's Butterflies of the Soul: Science and Art.* New York: Oxford University Press, 2009.

DeFelipe, Javier. "Cajal's Place in the History of Neuroscience." In *Encyclopedia of Neuroscience,* edited by Larry R. Squire. New York: Elsevier, 2009, pp. 497–507. doi:10.1016/B978-008045046-9.00989-X.

DeFelipe, Javier. "Sesquicentenary of the Birthday of Santiago Ramón y Cajal, the Father of Modern Neuroscience." *Trends in Neurosciences* 25, no. 9 (2002), 481–484. doi:10.1016/s0166-2236(02)02214-2.

DeFelipe, Javier. "The Dendritic Spine Story: An Intriguing Process of Discovery." *Frontiers in Neuroanatomy* 9 (March 5, 2015), 14. doi:10.3389/fnana.2015.00014.

DeFelipe, Javier, Eduardo Garrido, and Henry Markram. "The Death of Cajal and the End of Scientific Romanticism and Individualism." *Cell* 37, no. 10 (October 2014), 525–527. doi:10.1016/j.tins.2014.08.002.

DeFelipe, Javier and Edward G. Jones. "Santiago Ramón y Cajal and Methods in Neurohistology." *Trends in Neurosciences* 15, no. 7 (1992), 237–246. doi:10.1016/0166-2236(92)90057-f.

Domhoff, G. William. "Refocusing the Neurocognitive Approach to Dreams; A Critique of the Hobson Versus Solms Debate." *Dreaming* 15 (2005), 3–20. http://www2.ucsc.edu/dreams/Library/domhoff_2005b.html.

Dubos, René Jules and Jean Dubos. *The White Plague: Tuberculosis, Man, and Society.* New Brunswick, New Jersey: Rutgers University Press, 1952.

Dumas, Alexandre. *The Count of Monte Cristo,* translated by Peter Washington. New York: Knopf, 2009.

Ehrlich, Benjamin. "Santiago Ramón y Cajal: Café Chats." *New England Review* 33, no. 1 (2012).

El Sol, October 18, 1934, accessed from the Hemeroteca Digital, through Biblioteca Nacional de España, http://hemerotecadigital.bne.es/results.vm?q=parent%3A000 0182002&s=970&lang=en&t=-creation (accessed April 28, 2016).

Ellenberger, Henri F. *The Discovery of the Unconscious: The History and Evolution of Dynamic Psychiatry.* New York: Basic Books, 1970.

Espinosa, Lorena Desdentado. "Hipnosis en España desde la década de 1880 hasta 1936." http://www.elseminario.com.ar/biblioteca/Desdentado_Espinosa_Hipnosis_Espana.pdf.

Fereira, Francisco R. M., Javier DeFelipe, and Maria I. Noguiera. "The Influence of James and Darwin on Cajal and His Research into the Neuron Theory and Evolution of the Nervous System." *Frontiers in Neuroanatomy* 8, no. 1 (2014). doi:10.3389/fnana.2014.00001.

Fernandez Rodríguez, Juan. "Cajal–Freud: Vidas cruzadas." *Revista de Psicoterapia y Psicosomática* 30, no. 73 (2010), 9–12.

Freud, Sigmund. "Pre-Psychoanalytic Publications and Unpublished Drafts" vol. 1, "Early Psychoanalytic Publications" vol. 3, "The Interpretation of Dreams (1st Part)" vol. 4, and "The Interpretation of Dreams (2nd Part) and On Dreams" vol. 5. In *The Standard Edition of the Complete Psychological Works of Sigmund Freud,* translated from German under the general editorship of James Strachey, in collaboration with Anna Freud, assisted by Alix Strachey and Alan Tyson. London: Hogarth Press and the Institute of Psychoanalysis, 1953–1974.

"Freud's Book, 'The Interpretation of Dreams,' Released 1900." *A Science Odyssey: Peoples and Discoveries,* at PBS.org. http://www.pbs.org/wgbh/aso/databank/entries/dh00fr.html.

Frith, John. "History of Tuberculosis: Part 1—Phthsis, Consumption and the White." *Journal of Military and Veterans' Health* 22, no. 2 (June 2014), 29–35. http://jmvh.org/article/history-of-tuberculosis-part-1-phthisis-consumption-and-the-white-plague.

Fuentes, Manuel A. *Lima: Or Sketches of the Capital of Peru, Historical, Statistical, Administrative, Commercial, and Moral.* Paris: Firman Didot, Brothers, Sons & Co., 1866.

Fiorentini, Erna. "Inducing Visibilities: An Attempt at Santiago Ramón y Cajal's Aesthetic Epistemology." *Studies in History and Philosophy Part C: Studies in History and Philosopher of Biological and Biomedical Sciences* 42, no. 4 (December 2011), 391–394. doi:10.1016/j.shpsc.2011.07.008.

Garcia-Lopez, Pablo, Virginia Garcia-Marin, and Miguel Freire. "The Histological Slides and Drawings of Cajal." *Frontiers in Neuroanatomy* 4 (March 10, 2010). doi:10.3389/neuro.05.009.2010.

Gamundí, A., R. V. Rial, M. C. Nicolau, G. Timoner, and María Ángeles Langa. "La psicología sugestiva en Ramón y Cajal." *Revista de Historia de la Psicología* 16, nos. 3–4 (1995), 225–231. http://www.revistahistoriapsicologia.es/revista/1995-vol-16-n%C3%BAm-3-4.

Garcia-Lopez, Pablo, Virginia Garcia-Marin, and Miguel Freire. "The Histological Slides and Drawings of Cajal." *Frontiers in Neuroanatomy* 4, no. 9 (2010). doi:10.3389/neuro.05.009.2010.

Gay, Peter. *Freud: A Life for Our Time.* New York: Norton, 1988.

Glick, Thomas F. "The Naked Science; Psychoanalysis in Spain, 1914–1948." *Comparative Studies in Society and History* 24, no. 4 (1982), 533–571. http://isites.harvard.edu/fs/docs/icb.topic355408.files/Freud/Freud_Spain.pdf.

Goldman-Rakic, Patricia S. "The 'Psychic Cell' of Ramón y Cajal." *Progress in Brain Research* 136 (2002), 427–434. doi:10.1016/S0079-6123(02)36035-7.

Graus, Andrea. "Hypnosis in Spain (1888–1905): From Spectacle to Medical Treatment of Mediumship." *Studies in the Philosophy of Science Part C: Studies in History and Philosophy of Biological and Biomedical Sciences* 48 (2014), 85–93. doi:10.1016/j.shpsc.2014.07.002.

Haines, Duane E. "Santiago Ramón y Cajal at Clark University, 1899: His Only Visit to the United States." *Brain Research Reviews* 55, no. 2 (October 1, 2007), 463–480.

Hatzigiannakoglou, Paul D. and Lazaros C. Triarhou. "A Review of Heinrich Obersteiner's 1888 Textbook on the Central Nervous System by the Neurologist Sigmund Freud." *Wiener Medizinische Wochenschrift* 161, nos. 11–12 (2011), 315–325. doi:10.1007/s10354-011-0911-9.

Hippocrates. *On the Sacred Disease,* translated by Francis Adams. http://classics.mit.edu/Hippocrates/sacred.html.

"History of the Cajal Club," http://cajalclub.org/id3.html and a private conversation with a club member.

Hobson, J. Allan. *Dreaming and the Brain.* New York: Basic Books, 1989.

Sabourin, Michel and Saths Cooper. "The first International Congress of Physiological Psychology (Paris, August 1889): The birth of the International Union of Psychological Science." *International Journal of Psychology* 39, no. 3 (2014), 222–232. doi:10.1002/ijop.12071.

Jacobson, Marcus. *The Foundations of Neuroscience.* New York: Plenum, 1995.

"Jean-Martin Charcot: 1825–1893." *A Science Odyssey: People and Discoveries,* at PBS.org. http://www.pbs.org/wgbh/aso/databank/entries/bhchar.html.

Jones, Edward G. "Golgi, Cajal, and the Neuron Doctrine." *Journal of the History of Neuroscience* 8, no. 2 (1999), 170–178. doi:10.1076/jhin.8.2.170.1838.

Jones, Edward G. "Santiago Ramón y Cajal and the Croonian Lecture, March 1894." *Trends in Neurosciences* 17, no. 5 (1994), 190–192. doi:10.1016/0166-2236(94)90101-5.

Khan, M. Masud R. *Hidden Selves: Between Theory and Practice in Psychoanalysis.* London: Maresfield Library, 1988.

Køppe, Simo. "The Psychology of the Neuron: Freud, Cajal and Golgi." *Scandinavian Journal of Psychology* 24 (1983).

"La muerte de Don Santiago Ramón y Cajal." *Heraldo de Madrid,* October 18, 1934.

Lanfranco, Renzo C., Andrés Canales-Johnson, and David Huepe. "Hypnoanalgesia and the Study of Pain Experience: From Cajal to Modern Neuroscience." *Frontiers in Psychology* 5 (September 30, 2014), 1126. doi:10.3389/fpsyg.2014.01126.

Lanska, Douglas J. and Joseph T. Lanska. "Franz Anton Mesmer and the Rise of Animal Magnetism." In *Brain, Mind and Medicine: Neuroscience in the 18th Century,* edited by Harry Whitaker, C. U. M. Smith, and Stanley Finger. New York: Springer, 2007.

Letters of Sigmund Freud, translated by Tania and James Stern, edited by Ernst L. Freud. New York: Dover, 1992.

Littell, E. *Littel's Living Age.* Boston: Little and Company, 1852.

Lobato, R. D. "Historical Vignette of Cajal's Work 'Degeneration and Regeneration of the Nervous System' with a Reflection by the Author." *Neurocirugía* 19 (2008), 456–468. http://scielo.isciii.es/pdf/neuro/v19n5/8.pdf.

López-Ibor, J. J. "The Founding of the First Psychiatric Hospital in the World in Valencia." *Actas de Españolas Psiquiatría* 36, no. 1 (2008), 1–9.

López-Muñoz, Francisco, Cecilio Alamo, and Juan de Dios Molina Martín. "Los vínculos psiquisátricos en la obra y vida de Cajal." *Norte de Mental Salud: Revista de Salud Mental y Psiquitría Comunitaria* 8, no. 36 (2010). https://dialnet.unirioja.es/servlet/articulo?codigo=4830418.

López-Muñoz, Francisco, Gabriel Rubio, Juan D. Molina, Pilar García-García, Cecilio Álamo, and Joaquín Santo-Domingo. "Cajal y la Psiquiatría Biológica: El legado psiquiátrico de Ramón y Cajal (una teoría y una escuela)." *Archivos de Psiquiátria* 71, no. 1 (2008), 50–79. http://files.sld.cu/histologia/files/2012/04/08-historia-1-norte361.pdf.

López-Muñoz, Francisco, Jesús Boya, and Ceilio Alamo. "Neuron Theory, the Cornerstone of Neuroscience, on the Centenary of the Nobel Prize Award to Santiago Ramón y Cajal." *Brain Research Bulletin* 70, nos. 4–6 (2006), 391–405. doi:10.1016/j.brainresbull.2006.07.010.

López-Muñoz, Francisco, Jesús Boya, and Gabriel Rubio. "The Neurobiological Interpretation of the Mental Functions in the Work of Santiago Ramón y Cajal." *History of Psychiatry* 19, no. 1 (2008), 5–24. doi:10.1177/0957154x06075783.

López Piñero, José Maria. *Santiago Ramón y Cajal.* Valencia: Universitat de València, 2006.

Lothane, Zvi. "Freud's 1895 Project: From Mind to Brain and Back Again." *Annals of the New York Academy of Sciences* 843, no. 1 (1998), 43–65.

Madoz, Pascual. *Diccionario geográfico-estadístico-histórico de España y sus posesiones de Ultramar.* Madrid: 1845–1850.

"Madrid (From Our Regular Correspondent)." *Journal of the American Medical Association* 75, no. 6 (July 12, 1920).

Makari, George. *Revolution in Mind: The Creation of Psychoanalysis.* New York: Harper Perennial, 2009.

Marcus, Laura. "Introduction: Histories, Representations, Autobiographics in *The Interpretation of Dreams.*" In *The Interpretation of Dreams: New Interdisciplinary Essays,* edited by Laura Marcus. Manchester, UK: Manchester University Press, 1999.

Markel, Howard. *An Anatomy of Addiction: Sigmund Freud, William Halstead, and the Miracle Drug, Cocaine.* New York: Vintage Books, 2012.

Martinez, Alfredo, Virginia G. Marín, Santiago Ramón y Cajal Junquera, Ricardo Martínez-Murillo, and Miguel Freire. "The Contributions of Santiago Ramón y Cajal to Cancer Research—100 Years On." *Nature Reviews Cancer* 5 (November 2005), 904–909.

Merchan, Miguel A., Javier DeFelipe, and Fernando De Castro. *Cajal and de Castro's Neurohistological Methods.* New York: Oxford University Press, 2016.

Monasterio, Fernanda. "Las obras de José Germain." *Papeles de psicólogo,* nos. 28 and 29 (February 1982). http://www.papelesdelpsicologo.es/vernumero.asp?id=315.

Mora, Juan Antonio. "Semblanza Biográfica del Dr. D. José Germain Cebrián." *General de Colegios Oficiales de Psicólogos,* no. 70 (June 1998). http://www.cop.es/infocop/vernumeroCOP.asp?id=991.

Nature Magazine. "Human Brain Project Needs a Rethink." *Scientific American* (March 14, 2015). http://www.scientificamerican.com/article/human-brain-project-needs-a-rethink.

Nazarova, Maria and Evgeny Blagovechtchenski. "Modern Brain Mapping—What Do We Map Nowadays?" *Frontiers in Psychiatry* 6 (2015). doi:10.3389/fpsyt.2015.00089.

Nemri, Abdellatif. "Santiago Ramón y Cajal." *Scholarpedia* 5, no. 12 (2010), 8577. doi:10.4249/scholarpedia.8577.

Northoff, Georg. "Psychoanalysis and the Brain: Why Did Freud Abandon Neuroscience?" *Frontiers in Psychology* (April 2, 2012), 71. doi:10.3389/fpsyg.2012.00071.

Ochs, Sidney. *A History of Nerve Function: From Animal Spirits to Molecular Mechanisms.* Cambridge, UK: Cambridge University Press, 2004.

Otis, Laura. "Dr. Bacteria." *LabLit.com* (March 11, 2007). http://www.lablit.com/article/226.

Otis, Laura. *Membranes: Metaphors of Invasion in Nineteenth-Century Literature, Science, and Politics.* Baltimore, Maryland: Johns Hopkins University Press, 1999.

Otis, Laura. "Ramón y Cajal, a Pioneer in Science Fiction." *International Microbiology* 4, no. 3 (2001).

"People and Discoveries: Jean-Martin Charcot 1825–1893." *A Science Odyssey,* PBS.org. http://www.pbs.org/wgbh/aso/databank/entries/bhchar.html.

Piccolino, Marco, Enrica Strettoi, and Elena Laurenzi. "Santiago Ramón y Cajal, the Retina and the Neuron Theory." *Documenta Opthalmologica* 71, no. 2 (1989), 123–141. doi:10.1007/bf00163466.

Pintar, Judith and Steven J. Lynn. *Hypnosis: A Brief History.* Hoboken, New Jersey: Wiley-Blackwell, 2008.

Prioreschi, Plinio. "Possible Reasons for Neolithic Skull Trephining." *Perspectives in Biology and Medicine* 34, no. 2 (Winter 1991), 296–303.

Ramón y Cajal, Luis. "Cajal, as Seen by His Son." In *Proceedings of the Cajal Club* 4 (1996), edited by Duane E. Haines, 73. http://cajalclub.org/sitebuildercontent/sitebuilderfiles/cajalbk4chap15cajalasseebyhisson.pdf.

Ramón y Cajal, Pedro. "La juventud de Cajal contada por su hermano Don Pedro." In *La psicología de las artistas,* 3rd edition. Madrid: Espasa Calpe, S.A., 1972.

Ramón y Cajal, Santiago. *Advice for a Young Investigator,* translated by Neely Swanson and Larry W. Swanson, 1999.

Ramón y Cajal, Santiago. *Charlas de café,* 5th edition. Buenos Aires: Espasa Calpe, 1948.

Ramón y Cajal, Santiago. *El mundo visto a los ochenta años: Impresiones de un arteriosclerótico,* 5th edition. Buenos Aires: Espasa-Calpe, 1948.

Ramón y Cajal, Santiago. *La vida en el año 6000: Biblioteca Ramón y Cajal autografos de Cajal,* edited by García Durán Muñoz and Nana Ramón y Cajal de Durán. Cáceres, Spain: Tip. Extremadura, 1973.

Ramón y Cajal, Santiago. *Neuron Theory or Reticular Theory? Objective Evidence of the Anatomical Unity of Nerve Cells,* translated by M. Ubeda Purkiss and Clement A. Fox. Madrid: Consejo Superior de Investigaciones Científicas, Instituto Ramón y Cajal, 1951.

Ramón y Cajal, Santiago. *Obra literaria: Charles de café, Cuentos de vacaciones.* Zaragoza: Prames y Gobierno de Aragón, n.d.

Ramón y Cajal, Santiago. "Preface." In *Super-Organic Evolution: Nature and the Social Problem* by Enrique Lluria, translated by Rachel Challice. London: Forgotten Books, 2012.

Ramón y Cajal, Santiago. *Recollections of My Life,* translated by E. Horne Craigie with Juan Cano. Cambridge, Massachusetts: The MIT Press, 1989.

Ramón y Cajal, Santiago. *Trabajos escogidos.* Barcelona: Antoni Bosch, 2006.

Ramón y Cajal, Santiago. *Vacation Stories: Five Science Fiction Tales,* translated by Laura Otis. Urbana, Illinois: University of Illinois Press, 2005.

Ramón y Cajal Junquera, María Ángeles. "Santiago Ramón y Cajal y la hipnosis como anestesia." *Revista española de patología* 35, no. 4 (2002). http://www.patologia.es/volumen35/vol35-num4/35-4n07.htm.

Rizzuto, Anne-Marie. *Why Did Freud Reject God? A Psychodynamic Interpretation.* New Haven, Connecticut: Yale University Press, 1998.

Robin, Albert. "Treatment of Tuberculosis: Ordinary Therapeutics of Medical Men," translated by Dr. Léon Blanc. New York: Macmillan, 1913.

Rusiñol Estragués, Jordi and Virgili Ibarz Serrat. "La recepción del pensamiento de Freud en la obra de Ramón y Cajal." *Persona* 6 (2003), 75–80.

Saiz, Maria Dolores and Milgaros Saiz. *Personajes para una historia de la psicología en españa.* Madrid: Piramide, 1995.

Sala, José, Etzel Cardeña, María Carmen Holgado, Crióbal Añez, Pilar Pérez, Rocío Periñán, and Antonio Capafons. "The Contributions of Ramón y Cajal and Other Spanish Authors to Hypnosis." *Internation Journal of Clinical and Experimental Hypnosis* 56, no. 4 (2008), 361–372. doi:10.1080/00207140802255344.

Schore, Allan. "A Century After Freud's Project for Scientific Psychology: Is a Rapprochement Between Psychoanalysis and Neurobiology at Hand?" *Journal of the American Psychiatric Association* 45 (1997), 807–839.

Schwartz, Casey. *In the Mind Fields: Exploring the New Science of Neuropsychoanalysis.* Pantheon: New York, 2015.

Schwartz, Sophie. "A Historical Loop of One Hundred Years: Similarities Between 19th Century and Contemporary Dream Research." *Dreaming* 10, no. 1 (2000), 55–66. doi:10.1023/a:1009455807975.

Shepherd, Gordon. *Foundations of the Neuron Doctrine.* New York: Oxford University Press, 1991.

Sherrington, Charles. "A Memoir to Dr. Cajal." Introduction to *Explorer of the Human Brain,* by Dorothy Cannon. New York: Schuman, 1949.

Siegel, Lee. *Trance-Migrations: Stories of India, Tales of Hypnosis.* Chicago: University of Chicago Press, 2014.

"Sigmund Freud Chronology: 1895." Sigmund Freud Museum Vienna. http://www.freud-museum.at/online/freud/chronolg/1895-e.htm.

Simmons, Laurence. *Freud's Italian Journey.* Amsterdam: Rodopi, 2006.

Solms, Mark. "An Introduction to the Neuroscientific Works of Sigmund Freud." In *The Pre-Psychoanalytic Writings of Sigmund Freud,* edited by Gertrudis Van de Vijver Gertrudis and Filip Geeradyn. London: Karnac Books, 2002, pp. 17–35.

Sotelo, Constantino. "Viewing the Brain Through the Master Hand of Ramón y Cajal." *Nature Reviews Neuroscience* 4, no. 1 (2003), 71–77. doi:10.1038/nrn1010.

Stahnisch, Frank W. and Robert Nitsch. "Santiago Ramón y Cajal's Concept of Neuronal Plasticity: The Ambiguity Lives On." *Trends in Neurosciences* 25, no. 11 (2002), 589–591. doi:10.1016/s0166-2236(02)02251-8.

Stefanidou, Maria, Carme Solà, Elias Kouvelas, and Lazaros C. Triarhou. "Cajal's Brief Experimentation with Hypnotic Suggestion." *Journal of the History of the Neurosciences* 16, no. 4 (October 2007), 351–361.

Strachey, James. "Introduction." In *The Standard Edition of the Complete Psychological Works of Sigmund Freud*. London: Hogarth Press and the Institute for Psychoanalysis, 1953–1976.

Sulloway, Frank. *Freud, Biologist of the Mind: Beyond the Psychoanalytic Legend.* New York: Basic Books, 1970.

Swanson, Larry. "Preface to the American Translation." In *The Histology of the Nervous System in Man and Vertebrates*, translated by Neely Swanson and Larry W. Swanson. New York: Oxford University Press, 1991.

"The Cholera in Spain." *The New York Times* (June 20, 1890).

The Complete Letters of Sigmund Freud to Wilhelm Fliess, 1887–1904, edited by J. M. Masson. Cambridge, Massachusetts: Harvard University Press, 1985.

"The Young Physician." In *The Freud Encyclopedia: Theory, Therapy, and Culture*, by Edward Erwin. New York: Routledge, 2002.

Triarhou, Lazaros C. "A Review of Edward Flatau's 1894 Atlas of the Human Brain by the Neurologist Sigmund Freud." *European Neurology* 65, no. 1 (2011), 10–15. doi:10.1159/000322500.

Triarhou, Lazaros C. "Exploring the Mind with a Microscope: Freud's Beginnings in Neurobiology." *Hellenic Journal of Psychology* 6 (2009), 1–13.

Triarhou, Lazaros C. and Ana B. Vivas. "Cajal's Conjectures on the Psychology of Writers." *Perspectives in Biology and Medicine* 52, no. 1 (Winter 2008), 80–89. doi:10.1353/pbm.0.0069.

Triarhou, Lazaros C. and Manuel del Cerro. "Freud's Contribution to Neuroanatomy." *Archives of Neurology and Psychiatry* 42, no. 3 (March 1985), 282–287. doi:10.1001/archneur.1985.04060030104017.

"Tuberculosis in Europe and North America, 1800–1922." In *Contagion: Historical Views of Diseases and Epidemics*, from the Harvard University Library Open Collections Program. http://ocp.hul.harvard.edu/contagion/tuberculosis.html.

Van Hoorde, Hubert. "Freud's Merit as a Psychiatrist." In *The Pre-Psychoanalytic Writings of Sigmund Freud*, edited by Gertrudis Van de Vijver Gertrudis and Filip Geeradyn. London: Karnac Books, 2002.

Warshawsky, Rivka. "The Symptom as Metaphor: Freud's 'Project.'" In *The Pre-Psychoanalytic Writings of Freud*, edited by Gertrudis Van de Vijver Gertrudis and Filip Geeradyn. London: Karnac Books, 2002.

Yalom, Irvin D. *Existential Psychotherapy*. New York: Basic Books, 1980.

INDEX